WITHDRAWN
UTSA Libraries

AT ODDS
WITH AIDS

P9-ECN-522

RENEWALS 458-4574

ATE DUE

WITHDRAWN
UTSA Libraries

MERIDIAN

Crossing Aesthetics

Werner Hamacher

& David E. Wellbery

Editors

Translated by
Peter Gilgen and
Conrad Scott-Curtis

*Stanford
University
Press*

---

*Stanford
California
1996*

AT ODDS
WITH AIDS

Thinking and Talking
About a Virus

Alexander García Düttmann

Stanford University Press
Stanford, California

© 1996 by the Board of Trustees
of the Leland Stanford Junior University

Printed in the United States of America

CIP data appear at the end of the book

The publication of this work has been
subsidized by Inter Nationes, Bonn

'At Odds with AIDS:
Thinking and Talking About a Virus'
was originally published in German
in 1993 under the title
'Uneins mit AIDS: Wie über einen
Virus nachgedacht und geredet wird.'
© 1993 Fischer Taschenbuch Verlag GmbH,
Frankfurt am Main

Stanford University Press publications are
distributed exclusively by Stanford University
Press within the United States, Canada,
Mexico, and Central America; they are
distributed exclusively by
Cambridge University Press
throughout the rest of the world.

Library
University of Texas
at San Antonio

For L.

Hinterdrein ist es die Wunde selbst,
die ihn zwingt, *zu leben.*

(The very wound itself afterward compels
him *to live.*)

—Friedrich Nietzsche

Contents

Translators' Note

Alexander García Düttmann's main argument in *Uneins mit AIDS* centers around the German pun *uneins/un-eins*, which is impossible to render as comprehensible English in all its connotations. The standard *uneins* means disagreeing with, at odds with, or in opposition to something or someone, and we have translated it as "not-at-one." Analogously, we have rendered the author's nominalization *Uneins-sein* as "Being-not-at-one." Thus, to be not-at-one with AIDS means to take an oppositional stance toward the disease. Although opposition would seem to be the "natural" reaction to AIDS, García Düttmann is concerned with delineating the minimal requirements of effective opposition to the disease—both in the ways we talk and think about AIDS and in the ways we act individually and institutionally. The opposite of Being-not-at-one with AIDS, then, would be adjustment to, conciliation with, or acceptance of the disease, even to a point of agreement or identity, which is captured in the idiomatic German phrase *eins sein mit.*

But precisely the identity of *Eins-sein*, "Being-one," is at stake in the hyphenated neologism *un-eins*, meant to express lack of unity or coherence, difference from or non-identity with something. *Un-eins* and *Un-eins-sein* we have rendered as "not-one" and "Being-not-one," respectively. *Un-eins-sein mit AIDS*, "Being-not-one with AIDS," expresses not identifying (oneself) with AIDS, differing from the disease. In the time of AIDS, a fundamental Be-ing-not-one of the subject appears, that is, becomes visible: the constant threat of a death "before one's time" makes impossible the subject's full appropriation of a unified subjectivity. Thus, there is, in the author's words, always something "im-proper" in-habiting the subject. Therefore, attempts at creating subjectivity strictly along the lines of an identity politics, whether gay or oth-erwise, whether activist or strictly intellectual, are bound to fall short.

Analogous to the Being-not-one of the subject, the Being-not-one of time should be understood as an originary lack of coher-ence in time itself: any unity of historical time as epoch, any nar-rative coherence of time, is produced on a base that ultimately will not sustain such unity and such coherence in the face of the chal-lenge posed by a death that comes "before its time."

For the sake of the argument, it is important to keep in mind this distinction between "not-at-one" and "not-one," along with the complexity of their respective semantic fields. But the pun, the fact that these words are homophones, only distinguished by the graphic addition of a hyphen (which interrupts the unity of oppo-sition, of resistance expressed in *uneins*), also signifies that they must be fundamentally thought together, that resistance without the thinking of difference or non-identity has no merit or, rather, is not even truly possible.

We deviate from the conventions outlined here in only one case: the title of the book. An obvious reason for not choosing the ren-dering "Not (at) one with AIDS" is the unfamiliarity among an English-language readership with a semantic field that corresponds to the German *uneins* and the consequent opacity of such a title. However, there is also a strategic reason for our decision. Whereas the juxtaposition of "not-at-one" and "not-one" in the main body of the text stresses the philosophical question at stake in García Düttmann's essay, "At Odds with AIDS" brings out the more polemical and more activist connotations that are also part of the German *uneins mit*. In fact, the cover of the original German edi-tion reproduces a photograph by Brian Weil that depicts a confrontation between ACT UP activists and police in New York City. The tacit promise made is of a discussion of the possibilities of activism(s), of being against AIDS, of being at odds with AIDS. Thus, our title points to the political element in García Düttmann's discussion, while the main text upholds a consistent philosophical terminology. In this way, we hope to include the range of the semantic fields invoked in the German pun *uneins/un-eins*.

For similar reasons, we occasionally modified quotes from existing English translations whenever the context required it, or in order to achieve consistency within the works of authors translated by different translators (especially Heidegger and Kant), while in principle adhering to existing translations as closely as possible.

For this edition, the author added a number of passages. Furthermore, some elaboration of difficult points was included here and there, always with the author's consent. In addition, numerous passages were clarified in spoken communication with the author. Thus, this edition is not a direct translation of the German edition (1993) but in many places a reworking.

Two of the interjected personal narratives of the first chapter include unidentified quotes. The first, on page 9, is taken from Adorno's *Minima Moralia*, and the second, on page 21, is from Nietzsche's *Gay Science*.

Last but not least, we would like to take the opportunity to thank Letitia Scott-Curtis and Brooke Partridge for their support and their valuable editorial and stylistic suggestions. We also thank the author for his collaboration and Helen Tartar of Stanford University Press for being a patient and perceptive editor.

P.G. and C.S.-C.

AT ODDS
WITH AIDS

———————

§ 1 Dying Before One's Time

> To every thing there is a season, and a time to every purpose
> under the heaven;
> A time to be born, and a time to die; a time to plant, and a
> time to pluck up that which is planted;
> A time to kill, and a time to heal; a time to break down, and
> a time to build up;
> A time to weep, and a time to laugh; a time to mourn, and a
> time to dance;
> A time to cast away stones, and a time to gather stones
> together; a time to embrace, and a time to refrain from
> embracing;
> A time to get, and a time to lose; a time to keep, and a time
> to cast away;
> A time to rend, and a time to sew; a time to keep silence and
> a time to speak;
> A time to love and a time to hate; a time of war, and a time
> of peace.
>
> —Ecclesiastes 3.1–8

He is thrown into turmoil thinking about a death that could come any time in the next few years. And because he can't occupy himself with the certainty of dying, and in any case doesn't want to spend his time that way, he faces and makes me, almost his age, face the question of what it means to live with the certainty of death, of a death that can no longer be called, simply, indefinite. He is capable of imagining his own death; it is the thought of growing older that eludes him. As with all the other infected and the ill, the (social) distinction and stigma of the mark of AIDS affects every part of his life; he is forced and forces himself incessantly to observe his body, possible carrier of symptoms portending death. An expression of affliction and concern, the language used here always runs the risk of turning into jargon, a jargon of authenticity or interiority. But who will be surprised to read a book about AIDS that begins with these words? Words of resistance, of not wanting to occupy oneself with AIDS, of not being at one with AIDS;[1] words that also express fear of AIDS, a fear heightened by AIDS.[2]

In a study that emerged from clinical research, Martin Dannecker includes the following laconic explanation of "the anxiety about AIDS" homosexuals feel: "At its core, anxiety about AIDS consists of nothing but anxiety about dying before one's time" (Dannecker [1], p. 31). That the thought of a premature demise can indeed determine the way one reacts to the consequences of immune deficiency is confirmed by the statements of an actor who died in 1987. Tom Petchkiss was one of fifteen AIDS patients whose testimony and reports are included in Nicholas and Bebe Nixon's *People with AIDS*: "I feel betrayed. And I will die before I'm ready. 'Before my time,' isn't that what you say?" (Nixon and Nixon, p. 2) Anxiety because one has no more time to live and to die, because one no longer lives and has not yet died, because one has died already and nevertheless lives on, because life and death merge beyond recognition; anger because one cannot prepare in one's lifetime for the time of dying, because one has been betrayed and cheated not only out of one's life but also out of one's death, because one imagines oneself to be the victim of a life and a death that alternately occupy each other's position whenever one tries to grasp them, whenever one tries to orient oneself by means of their unavailable and nevertheless appointed time. ("To every thing there is a season. . . . ") One is not-one with AIDS to the degree that one is not-one with time, to the degree that one exists in the Being-not-one of time and that one is incapable of determining a measure of time that still permits the constitution of a lifetime.

Time won't tell: Is not the behavior of an infected person, for whom time seems to have nothing left in store but the outbreak of opportunistic diseases and finally a "premature" death, often marked by wavering, by doubting and questioning, by a split that makes it impossible for him or her to be in one place without at the same time being in another? Indifference, aimless circling within oneself, struggle against such indifference and circling; self-distraction and drifting, broken off by settling down, only to be interrupted again; sudden, defensive eruptions of hostility and violence; fatalism and surprising rapture. Is what is revealed in such fluctuation the splitting, the Being-not-one of time, the Being-not-one with AIDS that foils the constitution of a coherent time and of the coherence of a life? *Barely arrived in the city, he will warn him of his will to fate: his desire to have a fate, the desire of the unfortunate for misfortune, the desire of one who has no time but wants to manipulate this lack itself, by turning it into a fate. Time and again he will then speak of guilt, mostly in order to assert his innocence or to exonerate others from a fictional guilt. For example on that evening when he will tell him that he wants to convince the group of HIV-positive people and people with AIDS, which meets every Monday near his apartment, that none of them who infected a friend or a stranger without knowing his own status bears any guilt. But he who has no time, and who transmutes this lack into something he can handle by giving it the form of a fate, a fate that he vindicates as a fate and to which he submits, is guilty of closing himself off from others completely. In the fateful course of things, there is no time for otherness. Thus, fate carries only misfortune with it. Why does he want to have a fate? Why does he, asserting his innocence as one overtaken by fate, take guilt upon himself?* "Il est impossible de suivre ma trace, come celle du sida," *it is as impossible to follow my tracks as to follow the tracks of AIDS, says one who has dealt with originary contamination and contagion of the originary, with that which makes every trace into an arche-trace and thus leads the following of the trace onto an always new and inevitable detour: if AIDS, to which everybody can expose him- or herself at any time, no longer permits the following of traces, and thus perpetuates the question of contagion—Who infected me? Who infected the infected one who infected me?—then the desire to have a fate perhaps aims at the restitution of a narratable life story. By giving a form to his life, and thus submitting it to fate—as if he wanted to draw the map to which the ways of his life amount—he involuntarily turns it into the unchanging misfortune that erases every trace and in principle cannot be told, because in a life modeled according to fate nothing can happen anymore. He becomes guilty of a violation of life, which he be-*

lieves has become guilty of a violation of him, the infected one. And yet, in every instant he breaks free of the fate that he seems to submit to, and that he seems to impose upon himself; his words and gestures were always hedged with uncertainty and hesitation, a Being-not-at-one with the fateful Being-not-one, and they continue to be so, and that is why you love him.

The Being-not-one of time as Being-not-one with AIDS represents the collapse of the subject, through and for which the unity of life exists. What does it mean if the concept of a lifetime turns out to be useless for the purpose of describing experience as the unified experience of a subject? What does it mean if there is no more time for life and for death, if the experience of time, which is no longer part of a coherent and continuous time, becomes merely the impossible and untimely experience of a before-one's-time, of an originary alienation? Is it possible to be not-at-one with AIDS while appealing to a lost temporal unity, which is also the unity of space and time? (Lifetime and city: New York or San Francisco as metropolis of a "past" way of life and emblematic site of the epidemic.) Is it possible to be not-at-one with AIDS while lamenting this lost unity, while not really measuring up to the demands of the Being-not-one of time?

We might try to anchor existence in the unity of time, to tie it back into the unity of time[3]—into the unity of life's coherence that extends from birth to death and is coherent only insofar as everything out of its proper time can, in the end, be integrated into life's connectedness—even if only as a negative complement, an incomprehensible interruption and reminder of the unavailability of closure ("To every thing there is a season . . . "). But this "tying back into," along with any appeal to feelings of anxiety and anger, which are themselves marked by a presupposed coherence of life, necessarily justifies AIDS, more specifically Being-not-one with AIDS, even if the intent is exactly opposite. And this justification conceals Being-not-one with AIDS, just as it disguises the Being-not-one of time, and must be understood as playing down the consequences of immune deficiency, and thus as having the effect of prolonging helplessness in the face of these consequences.

In other words, if it is correct that anxiety about AIDS and the anger caused by AIDS can be traced back to loss of the time one has to live, to the destruction of a meaningful, unified coherence in which living and dying have their time, then one can respond to their reactive character neither by positing as permanent the mourning of the loss—of one's own living and dying—nor by attempting to restore the Being-one of time and constituting a subject with AIDS. Further, the inadequacy of such responses holds not only for the period during which a drug to fight AIDS has not yet been discovered and successfully tested. If the destruction of time, of what we call lifetime, must be counted among the consequences of this pandemic, one is obliged to take into account the *possibility* of such a threat whether or not one successfully brings to bear a vaccine against AIDS. How else could one explain what it is that has determined the transformation of AIDS into a paradigm, a paradigm of the contemporary social-economic-political-technical state of the western world, which necessarily includes its relationship to other worlds, to other continents and countries?[4] If we go back to the difficulties of constituting the unity of time and a unified subject in order to understand why AIDS becomes a paradigm of the present, we recognize that AIDS becomes a sign: it takes on an indicative value, one unappreciated by the restituting intention, or one that the restituting intention recognizes only too well. But is not the indicating of a paradigm—both the pointing out of a paradigmatic model and the indicating function carried out by the paradigm itself—a gesture of restitution, of generalization, of universalization, of unification of time? Is there a diagnosis of time that does not annul Being-not-one with AIDS? *And every time they mention the transportation and communication systems in order to emphasize the specifically "modern" character of the epidemic, he thinks of a fax, in the middle of the night in a Spanish hotel room, early in the morning in a North American apartment or in a French post office, liaison, he never liked the word but accepted it nevertheless, like everything that came from him, between all the cities and languages. But he also thinks of the portraits, the facsimiles of the artist who volunteered his works for the English publication, and whose boyfriend he met in New York. He had just returned from a conference. They owe their existence to fax transmissions, "the Proud Lives to which these likenesses recall the viewer are those of men now dead, commemorated in a regular feature of that title in the Toronto bi-weekly* Xtra!, *which publishes the photographs of members of the community recently lost to AIDS-related illness. . . . Because Andrews was absent from Toronto, away from home and community (and his usual locus of production) when the photographs ran in* Xtra!, *he first received the images via transatlantic fax."*

What is a sign that shows itself as a sign, and at the same time crosses itself out, because it must remain, finally, without mean-

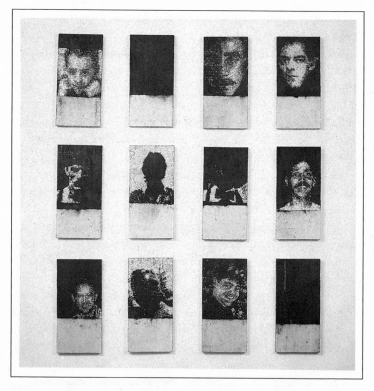

Fig. 1 Stephen Andrews, *Picture with Juxtaposed "Facsimiles"*

ing, because it does not refer to a meaning and therefore cannot be the sign of a meaning, not even the sign of a complementary meaninglessness, of a sudden, unexpected demise that unhinges the order of things and can be interpreted either as a flaw or as a reminder of repressed death?[5] Martin Dannecker chooses as a title for his book, *The Homosexual Man Under the Sign of AIDS*. The therapeutic orientation of the sexologist essentially determines his understanding AIDS as the sign of a (missing) meaning and makes understanding his title dependent on such a perception. His approach becomes particularly clear when a reconstruction of the psychoanalytically decoded life history and the "valorization of homosexuality" connected with it are supposed to remedy "anxiety about AIDS": "It seems to me that from these life-historical experiences, only crudely outlined and unduly schematized here, a way leads to the understanding of the specific conflicts in which homosexual men often get involved when they hear that they are infected with HIV or ill with AIDS. AIDS evokes earlier feelings of rejection, shame, and inferiority and is experienced as a punishment for being different and for the forbidden desire directed toward the father. It is obvious that in light of such massive internal conflicts even the slightest threat of punishment by outside authorities against people infected with HIV and ill with AIDS can cause a severe psychic crisis. There is no other way to overcome such a crisis than by a valorization of homosexuality by others, that is, a 'revaluation' of what is experienced as abominable. That can happen in the course of psychotherapy, or in self-help groups, or elsewhere" (Dannecker [1], pp. 91–92). If AIDS is thus turned into the sign of a (missing) meaning, it is inevitable that the therapy required because of the lack (of a meaning) reproduces anxiety about dying "before one's time," at least virtually.

How exactly the (missing) meaning can be acquired is not always immediately clear in Dannecker. In his study of AIDS and homosexuality, meaning is guaranteed by the reconstruction and revaluation of the life history undertaken in psychotherapy or in "self-help groups." But if we turn to an earlier text, to an interview with Rosa von Praunheim published in 1987, the acquisition or reappropriation of the (missing) meaning is presented in a more contradictory way. Here, Dannecker claims that its possibility depends on mourning the loss of a life characterized by promiscuity. Such mourning alone is supposed to confer meaning on the process of reflection and enlightenment, which can be used to combat the anxiety brought on by an unmediated transition from one way of life to another, entirely different one: "In these safer sex brochures, especially when they display an American influence, safe sex is always represented as something incredibly wild, or else it is simply demanded. No issue is made of the change and adaptation being required here, and of the fact that something like that always produces anxiety" (Dannecker [2], p. 92). What should be mourned, though? Promiscuity—which in principle must not be mourned because "the tendency to promiscuity among homosexuals" is supposed to have something to do "with narcissistic disharmonies" (p. 94) and cannot be elevated to a (sexual) ideal? Here, reflection and enlightenment have as their own condition the paradoxical construct of an objectless mourning that always already mourns itself.

AIDS is the sign of a (missing) meaning because only AIDS paves the way to this meaning. But of course this process brings with it the danger that anxiety might rob reflection and enlightenment of time: "How much time do you have for it?" asks Praunheim. Praunheim, who himself puts too much trust in the irrationality of an anxiety that functions in the service of securing an identity ("and I'm doing awfully well this way"), reproaches Dannecker for recommending reactive behavior. For Dannecker, the necessity of renunciation leads to mournful involvement in a restrictive sexual praxis rather than being actively accepted. Praunheim denounces the justification of an unhappy consciousness and body, a justification that for the enlightener—or the "subject under the sign of AIDS"—necessarily consists of a double demand, the demand for renunciation and a more or less free decision to choose or avoid the heightened risk.[6] However, the fact that both recommendation and justification presuppose an interpretation remains hidden: they become possible only after AIDS is interpreted as a sign of a (missing) meaning.

Wherever AIDS arouses anxiety about dying "before one's time," wherever it provokes anger about the interruption of the time of a life that no longer presents its natural and meaningful end, in short, wherever AIDS becomes the sign of a (missing) meaning, and the possibility of living under such a sign is given, the consciousness of that anxiety or that anger, as well as the reflexivity through which one experiences oneself as living under the sign of AIDS, must raise the question of whether one's own behavior did not also determine the loss or the lack of a coherent meaning of life and death. This question is the question of guilt. It is the question of conscience. Even the slogan "All people with AIDS are innocent," aimed at physicians and intended as a social critique, reminds us of this question. The slogan announced the Spring AIDS Action 1988 in the United States and was meant as an attack on the distinction between guilty and innocent AIDS "victims" as perpetuated by the media (Crimp and Rolston, p. 57). Isn't it really the tendency of the certainty and definiteness of death to coincide that sets up the possibility of seeing oneself as guilty and condemned, as someone struck by a curse or overtaken by fate because of one's guilt? Doesn't fate deliver the guilty over into a time that passes without their being able to make use of it? *The Body Positive: your love is your guilt you love your virus because you must submit to it as to all the bodies that must not love you to be loved by all these bodies you have kept back the virus that makes you cringe at night in your sleep every jerk every thrust reminds you of one of the forgotten bodies that gather in the park at the river and prolong the night of your love from which you have wanted to protect me since that day of which your name is the imperfect anagram in the other language:* "Truly terrifying are the sleepless nights when time seems to contract and run fruitlessly through our hands. . . . In a similar way the condemned man may see his last moments slip away unarrested, unused. But what is revealed in such contraction of the hours is the opposite of time fulfilled. If in the latter the power of experience breaks the spell of duration and gathers past and future into the present, in the hurried, sleepless night duration causes unendurable dread. Man's life becomes a moment, not by sublating duration but by decaying into nothingness, waking to its own futility in face of the bad infinity of time itself."

In his text *My AIDS*, Jean-Paul Aron claims that AIDS allows him to come to himself, to return to himself, that it leads him (back) to himself. Self-knowledge and the acquisition of what is supposed to make it possible coincide: in knowing oneself by means of AIDS, one appropriates it. Only AIDS makes one admit or acknowledge something; admission and acknowledgment amount to self-knowledge. But self-knowledge transforms AIDS into one's own AIDS. Is not anxiety about AIDS perhaps also anxiety that the Being-not-one of time might make such an appropriation more difficult? *My AIDS*: with this text the author publicly and contentiously admits his disease and his homosexuality. More precisely, he publicly admits it *to himself*. If AIDS effects a return to oneself, every admission of the infection or disease is an admission *to oneself*, a making sure of oneself, an awakening through which one becomes aware of oneself. Aron turns *himself* against those intellectuals who, it seems to him, are taken aback by an aggressive admission. The text also contains a confession that calls truth and thus conscience by name: every confession of AIDS is truly a confession only to the extent that the virus lets the one who confesses come to himself. Whoever speaks in the name of truth, and confesses himself to himself, must not be guided by a conscience that might allow false feelings of guilt to arise. "Today, when I have come to the decision to speak the truth, I confess that I do not in retrospect feel any remorse at the thought of having infected other people—at a time, to be sure, when I did not yet know that I carried a virus in me" (Aron, p. 24). The confessional mode and the invocation of knowledge and truth come as no surprise here. It is well known that autobiographical discourse, the retrospective view of one's own lifetime, of one's own life history, often determines the discourse on AIDS, whether or not it is a

matter of a challenge and a reaffirmation[7] of a claim, and whether
or not conversion and remorse are expressed.[8]

The sociologist Michael Pollak confirms these observations in
his description of the tone and style of the interviews he conducted
during his survey of homosexuality and AIDS: "In general one
finds in these interviews the main features of literary autobiography: its intimate character, its references to a lost paradise, to
happy days gone by, and to moments of conversion" (Pollak, p.
16). Undoubtedly, one must ask whether recourse to the genre of
autobiography is *typical* or *indicative* of the way homosexuals talk
about AIDS. But what conclusion is one supposed to draw from
the fact that AIDS provides the occasion for autobiographical reflection, for witnessing, admitting, confessing? The British author
Alan Hollinghurst considered a different ending to his successful
novel, *The Swimming-Pool Library* (1988), in which, probably for
reasons of historical accuracy, AIDS is not mentioned: the young
guy who lives in Holland Park and never stops cruising would
have told his story from his deathbed, suffering from AIDS. *One
always confesses without really knowing what one confesses to whom
one confesses something for how could one know to whom one confesses
something if one does not really know what one confesses one does not
even know that one confesses to oneself that is to the other I don't know
what I say when I turn to you unconscious confession is what the psychoanalyst calls it is there a need for punishment on the part of the infected or sick person who openly confesses for the psychoanalyst an open
confession marked as such can only be one degree of the forms an unconscious confession assumes which is all there is in the end by the way
confession resembles safer sex where anxiety is directed toward confession where confession satisfies the need for punishment it is comparable
to the fore-pleasure that replaces intercourse all forms of expression are
forms of expression of the unconscious confession because an absolutely
free uninhibited expression cannot exist at all an expression that does
not already encounter resistance in the instant of its utterance of its
coming to language and only thus becomes expression that is unconscious confession the smallest shortest distance between the expression*

and the fulfillment is sufficient to restrain and to impede it pure ex-
pression and metalanguage confession in which what is confessed be-
comes absolutely transparent and brought to consciousness coincide so
that there is only the infinite insatiable need for deciphering that can
be fulfilled only incompletely you want to decipher this unconscious
confession I put down in your large notebook between names addresses
phone and flight numbers dates and times balances appointments also
my name my address my phone number I wrote down in it on that
Sunday when I flew back and you accompanied me to 79th Street since
the need for the deciphering of the need can never be satisfied and Be-
ing-not-one never ceases perhaps nothing is more urgent than the trans-
formation of the impediment and of Being-not-one I do not know
what to whom I confess but I always also do something different than
invite you to decipher do it.

Challenge or transformation: the necessity of confession, which
is never of purely informative value, makes clear that the diagnosis
of AIDS—or the diagnosis of HIV infection—poses not only the
question of treatment but also a question of guilt and blindness.
Even if not knowing serves to justify lack of remorse and feelings
of guilt, the loss of innocence, of certainty, of conviction, of faith,
of confidence, of trust, retrospectively affects what is lost. There is
no pure loss. There is no loss without contagion and contamination and without loss of the loss.

Thus, it becomes evident why confession—for example, the
confession of having become sick with AIDS—always comes
across as *urgent testimony*. "The desire to bear witness becomes increasingly urgent. Perhaps in this way I try to follow the rhythm of
the virus shaking and unsettling my head and my body." These
are the first words of an autobiographical report that appeared in
the French daily *Libération* on November 15, 1990. It appeared under the (perhaps ironic) title "My AIDS and I," in a column where
Pierre Chablier, HIV-positive since 1988, regularly gives testimony
of the state of his health. In the instant that I decide to tell the
truth, to speak the truth (paradoxically enough, the measure of
truth is precisely this resolution, my decision),[9] in the instant I talk
about my AIDS and in its name, credible because I confess (to my-

self) my disease or contagion, I throw myself onto the virus, I run after it, I begin to be guided by it, to follow it, to love it and to hate it, as if I were one of the survivors of an impending apocalypse, one of those children who, in Joseph Losey's film *The Damned*, are immune to radioactivity because a radioactive womb conceived them. Only in the end do they understand their difference from all others. But is it not the experience of their flight from the place of their lifelong imprisonment that eventually makes them love and hate their cold, dead, living-dead bodies? *They seem to understand everything you too cannot always resist the temptation when for example they talk about a self-destructive urge about a perverse wish or about a fascination with death about the magical attempt to transcend AIDS how could I have loved you without loving more and more your saliva your semen your sweat your tears and thus the virus in your body yes I confess all the secretions you gave me little poisoned gifts I must love them no chance.*

The admission, the confession, the urgent testimony that express contagion make it possible to survive oneself in language: perverse purification that consists of contagion. Through this purification one escapes a death "before one's time," even if the purification does not simply renew the time of life, its meaningfully unified coherence. If I refuse to talk about AIDS without confessing my AIDS, if I do not want to talk about myself any longer without talking about my AIDS, I am already my own survivor, I am already another in myself, a mutant. I have survived myself: "Sometimes I have the feeling that we are tens of thousands of mutants in the midst of the crowd here in Paris," notes the witness who reports on "his" AIDS in *Libération*.

But it would be overly reductive to recognize in this admission and confession merely the survival strategy of a purification through contagion. First and foremost they seem to increase the destructive effects of the virus, and credit AIDS, make a reputation for AIDS, a reputation to which the one who confesses falls victim. In the novel *To the Friend Who Did Not Save My Life* (1990), the first part of a trilogy that centers around a protagonist suffering from AIDS, Hervé Guibert writes: "But the admission [gave rise to something terrible]: to say that one was sick only re-inforced the disease [*ne faisait qu'accréditer la maladie*], which sud-denly became real, quite remorseless, and seemed to draw its power and destructive force from whatever control it was granted [*du crédit qu'on lui accordait*]" (Guibert [1], p. 148/164). A confession is necessarily an affirmation, no matter how else one behaves toward the thing confessed. By confessing AIDS, one promotes AIDS. One feeds the virus to oneself and weakens the immune system for a second time: "It is said that each reintroduction of the AIDS virus through bodily fluids—blood, sperm, tears—renews the at-tack on the already infected patient" (Guibert [1], p. 4/12).

This is his secret. He discloses it to me because it binds him—be-cause his disclosure and betrayal bind him to me forever. He hadn't told anyone what I confided to him, as if it were my secret, and yet suddenly he told everyone. He couldn't talk to anyone without telling him, not because he wanted to betray me, but because the highest loy-alty he was capable of could consist only of spreading what was con-fided to him. It could consist only of such an immense scattering, of such an enormous betrayal that the unsayable, that is, the only thing that one can admit to, had to lose its magic power, "le sida . . . aura été un paradigme dans mon projet de dévoilement de soi et de l'énoncé de l'indicible," AIDS will have been a paradigm in my project of self-revelation and the formulation and speaking of the unsayable. Without AIDS I can neither experience nor learn what it means to disclose my being and to come back to myself. He wanted to free me from the power of confession. I should no longer be bound to the catastrophe of the secret, as I still was during that night I confided it to him, tired from the flight and shortly before we went to bed.

Guibert's novels contain the two decisive topoi of self-reflection, which continually recur and which the virus triggers in varying modifications. The first is the topos of coming to oneself under the sign of AIDS, by means of which dying "before one's time" is turned into its opposite and AIDS becomes the paradigm of the time of living and dying, of the coherent life story that can be told or narrated. AIDS is the ("modern") paradigm of all paradigmatic situations,[10] if paradigmatic situations can come about only where a well-defined time is given and a definite unity can be produced: "It is an illness with steps, a long staircase that leads with certainty to death, and whose every step represents a specific apprenticeship. It is an illness that grants one time to die, that gives death time to live: time to discover time and finally to discover life. It is, as it were, an ingenious modern invention, bequeathed to us by the African green monkey" (Guibert [1], p. 164/181). AIDS, paradigm of coming to oneself, thus appears as a paradoxical experience of a bound of time, which alone allows us to discover the time of living and dying: Being-one with AIDS, with Being-not-one, the living of death as an elimination of borders, a de-limitation that permits the circumscription of life and death.

The second topos of self-reflection becomes evident as a problematic of writing: in the short time left, the sick person who attempts to come to himself through writing must write all the books that remain to him to be written. But time for writing, the time that actually corresponds to these books, is being robbed by death, by the fact that the author will die "before his time." Writing devours the time it no longer has, since it is devoured by time and since Being-not-one threatens to cancel the production of coherence and unity. Because the paradigmatic experience is always self-contradictory and self-exclusive, not-one with itself, Guibert's novels also contain the topos of Being-not-one and Being-not-at-one. "This book, which tells the story of my fatigue, makes me forget it," writes Guibert. He continues, "and at the same time each phrase torn from my brain, which will be threatened by the intrusion of the virus once the tiny lymphatic belt gives out, only makes me want more than ever to close my eyes" (Guibert [1], p. 58/67). Elsewhere, Being-not-one is generalized and is related to (incurable) illness in general: "I don't know what to think about any of these crucial questions, about this alternation of certain death and sudden reprieve. . . . I tell myself that this book's *raison d'être* lies only along this borderline of uncertainty, so familiar to all sick people everywhere" (Guibert [1], pp. 2–3/10–11). However, Being-not-one—and Being-one with Being-not-one—leads finally to a Being-not-at-one with Being-not-one, with AIDS; the discovered time and the wisdom of discovery have their own time: they are finite. Guibert writes, "Certainly, I've had to love it, otherwise my life would have become unlivable; it has inevitably been a fundamental, crucial experience, but now that I've been through it all, I can't go any further. After that long road toward wisdom a revolt is stirring in me for the first time. I now can't bear any talk of AIDS. I hate AIDS. I want to have done with it, it's served its time in me" (Guibert [3], p. 42/64).

But if admitting and confessing—which can be urgent testifying or a survival strategy of purification through contagion, through self-poisoning—do not exhaust themselves in any of these causes, effects, and modes of action, it is also due to another reason. The Spanish philosopher María Zambrano points to the essence of admission and confession when she maintains that they are tied to the expectation that that which is not already part of oneself might come into appearance (Zambrano, p. 22). In our context, it is perhaps less important to feature, as Zambrano does, the production or the appearance of unity, in which one's own imperfection (the "fragmentary character of all life," as she calls it) finds its complement, than to emphasize a certain Being-not-one. This Being-not-one lies in the expectation of a manifestation of truth and perfection, where expectation takes the form of an admission or a confession. Even when there is a time to live and a time to die ("To every thing there is a season . . . "), even when the unity and coherence of life seem to be preserved, and death still has the meaning of a measure, time, insofar as it is allowed you, is not at your disposal. Anyone who had control over the time of living and dying would actually have no time to live and to die: the time of a life never just forms a closed unity and always already exposes itself to Being-not-one. AIDS as a diagnosis—which is more than just a diagnosis because it leads to the decision to confess (to oneself)—exposes, in the course of all appropriations and manifestations of unity, the Being-not-one of time and the self, and sets off the impossible experience of this Being-not-one, experience of the uncertainty of all bounds and limits. The existence of a person who is HIV-positive or diagnosed with AIDS is therefore defined by the way he or she relates to this Being-not-one. Existence exhibits Being-not-one even at the moment that resolute coming to oneself, or psychotherapeutic reconstruction of a life history, or integration into a (politically active) community of affected people attempts to consolidate Being-one—that is, attempts to consolidate a uniform coherence of life, a new-old identity. *All the names of the dead as if the community that calls itself the AIDS community were based on the memory of names they all want to be connected by an unmediated memory transmission as soon as another name is added to the list they know immediately like you when you were moved to speak on our walk at the shore by the death of the other you heard about only three days after "because we won't let them forget" what else am I doing but working on a text-quilt I weave only one name into the carpet you are my faith and therefore the indubitable reason for my doubts your decision for a death before death a decision that delivers me into undecidability between a natural and an artificial memory—did all this happen—your forgetting which sustains the soul's formation does not give me a choice mourning and calling over and over again remain in my love wrap yourself in these words burn them so that we can breathe nothing shall disclose nothing silence my song maybe you brought me death so that I write all this three thousand miles away from you and three hours younger even today it is impossible for me to think without counting the hours that separate our lives I had to wait until day broke in your city how often did I wake up in the middle of the night a prisoner of my sleep condemned to immobility in a world I couldn't share with you because in the end I had to succumb to fatigue you made me love the asynchronicity that suffocates me thus you become the witness of your own disappearance and thus you recollect yourself in me "any remembrance is appropriate" it says in a brochure of the NAMES Project AIDS Memorial Quilt in October nineteen hundred ninety-two the quilt weighs thirty-two tons and is exhibited in Washington "a San Francisco Group, whose work has now become national and has been shown in many cities, created a giant quilt containing hundreds of*

panels in memory of those who have died of AIDS, thus both 'indi-
vidualizing' persons with AIDS and allowing members of the com-
munity (and even those not directly connected with it) to share and
express their grief and anguish."

Is the Being-not-one of time and the self, which is exposed in
each attempt to appropriate and consolidate a uniform coherence
of life, comparable to the "dispersion," "disconnectedness," and
"inauthentic historicality" from which, if one follows the existential analytic, the very question of the connectedness of life [*Leben-
szusammenhang*] arises? Heidegger wants to make clear that the
question of the unity of Dasein and of its life, which "stretches
along" between birth and death, persists as long as Dasein perse-
veres irresolutely in the "disconnectedness" of "dispersion" and
"inauthentic historicality." He speaks, in the formal terms of phe-
nomenology, of a " 'natural' horizon for such questions" and emphasizes that "the origin of this question betrays that it is an inap-
propriate one if we are aiming at a primordial existential interpretation of Dasein's totality of historizing." "Everyday Dasein," he
writes, "has been dispersed into the many kinds of things which
daily 'come to pass.' . . . It is driven about by its 'affairs.' So if it
wants to come to itself it must first *pull itself together* from the *dispersion* and *disconnectedness* of the very things that have 'come to
pass'; and because of this, it is only then that there at last arises
from the horizon of understanding which belongs to inauthentic
historicality, the *question* of how one is to establish a 'connectedness' of Dasein if one does so in the sense of 'experiences' of a subject—experiences which are 'also' present-at-hand. The possibility
that this horizon for the question should be the dominant one is
grounded in the irresoluteness which goes to make up the essence
of the self's in-constancy" (Heidegger [1], p. 442/390). Here Heidegger presents the decisive argument concerning the question of
the unifying "connectedness" of life, which is supposed to free the
vision of dying "before one's time" of its dispersive effects. The belatedness that is constitutive of this question condemns to futility
every attempt at unifying what is dispersed. If one is satisfied with
juxtaposing a new-old identity or totality against the "disconnect-

edness" engendered by AIDS, one has already given in to the dispersion and become, as Heidegger says quoting Nietzsche, "too old for one's victories."[11] The argument of the belatedness, the reactivity of any attempt to establish an identity or totality out of the "disconnectedness" engendered by AIDS is not invalidated just because Being-not-one with AIDS might lend itself to being characterized in terms of "inauthenticity" and "lostness" in "the they" [*das Man*], but not in terms of the "authentic Being-toward-death" that is adopted in "resoluteness against the inconstancy of dispersion" and signifies the possibility "of existing as total potentiality for Being." At least, such an assertion can be made if one ascribes to AIDS a relevance that is not exhausted in the ontic-historical.

One loses oneself in "everyday concern," in distraction, and in "being driven about," only to pose, time and again, the question of the connectedness of life. The double movement characteristic of dispersed Dasein describes, equally well, the movement of a Dasein not-one with AIDS. The comparison, however, is not really valid. Since "inauthenticity is based on the possibility of authenticity," "everyday Being-toward-death" remains linked to the certainty and indefiniteness of death: both reveal their true nature in the anticipation of the "indefinite certainty of death." Dasein that has fallen into the "idle talk of the day" acknowledges only "something like a *certainty* of death" and confines itself "to conceding the 'certainty' of death in this ambiguous manner": "One says, 'death certainly comes, but not right away.' . . . Thus the 'they' covers up what is peculiar in death's certainty—*that it is possible at any moment.* Along with the certainty of death goes the *indefiniteness* of its 'when.' Everyday Being-toward-death evades this indefiniteness by conferring definiteness upon it. But such a procedure cannot signify calculating when the demise is due to arise. In the face of definiteness such as this, Dasein would sooner flee. Everyday concern makes definite for itself the indefiniteness of certain death by interposing before it those urgencies and possibilities which can be taken in at a glance, and which belong to the everyday matters that are closest to us" (Heidegger [1], p. 302/258). Certainty and indefiniteness go together: death is certain *because* it is indefinite, because it can arrive at any moment. If death were definite for Dasein, it could not live in its certainty, for certainty requires a peculiar indefiniteness that does not exclude the definite, the possibility of making the indefinite definite. Without this indefiniteness we would be set blindly before the inevitable and the definite; we would be exposed to them helplessly; and not even be "certain" of them. Without indefiniteness, everyday Dasein could not evade and flee that which is certain.[12] Only a certain and therefore indefinite death makes possible the covering up of certainty, which is effected by turning indefiniteness into definiteness. (Dasein represses or covers up the indefiniteness of certain death not simply by replacing it with definiteness, with things that can be defined. For this repressing or covering up consists of making the indefinite itself definite.) One can "confer definiteness" upon the indefinite only inasmuch as one could die at any moment, inasmuch as dying becomes most everyday and even most definite. And one can define the indefinite only inasmuch as death, in the end, dissolves and disappears in its own indefiniteness.[13] The essential belonging together of certainty and indefiniteness is virtually already a covering up of that which belongs together.

It would seem that the comparison between Being-not-one with AIDS and the dispersion of Dasein is limited because one must not confuse the defining of the indefinite with the tendency of certainty and definiteness to coincide. It is this latter tendency that plunges Dasein into the turmoil of dying "before one's time," a turmoil characterized by anxiety and anger. If it is true that one must not confuse Being-not-one with AIDS with the dispersion of Dasein, if it is true that Being-not-one with AIDS is not just another form of the dispersion of Dasein, perhaps this distinction should be understood as an indication that the "existential projection of an authentic Being-toward-death" itself experiences a limitation: the entire existential analytic of Dasein is affected. Or is it just a question here of spectacular exceptions and special cases, of an interruption that in the final analysis is only short term and not really representative? Does Being-not-one with AIDS just give the appearance of complete upheaval, which will last only until the day a vaccine is found and a person who is HIV-positive or has AIDS will have survived? Are we giving too much importance in this description of Being-not-one to a destructive *coincidence* of certainty and definiteness? Is not the indefiniteness that makes it impossible to know the precise hour of one's death sufficient to make us see this description of Being-not-one as undue emphasis, as exaggeration, as dramatization that dispossess the malady of its gravity by burdening it with excessive weight? What, though, becomes of the specific stretch of time during which people are not-one with AIDS if one considers that anyone at any time anywhere could contract the infection or infect another? What becomes of it if one considers that AIDS prescribes restrictive rules of behavior for all humankind and touches everyone without exception—not just a section of the population, an identifiable, isolated group? What becomes of it if one considers that in the end no spatially or temporally organized control could be sufficient, no quarantine comprehensive enough?

Anonymity preserved by an assigned number and a proper name attended by all the friends who consider me heedless who warned me about it and urged me to do it who could not understand that I didn't spend sleepless nights and that I felt almost ashamed to force a repetition of the ever-same scene on the friendly Polish doctor these cheap theatrics one calls the moment of truth where does AIDS paranoia start where does it end AIDS dementia is an imprecise term clinicians and researchers use for diagnostic and surveillance purposes in order to forget this barely tolerable scene repression they will think you however recall the two verses "Only now you're truly well / Those are well who have forgotten" I ventured into a conversation with the doctor I wanted to find out what science knows about side-effects of your AZT therapy imagine several times a day it enters your mind.

Death is the paradoxical possibility of the impossibility of Dasein; it is from this perspective that we must think totality—totality as a mode of being by which Dasein distinguishes itself. Totality's inauthentic form—a connectedness of life always yet-to-be-produced and therefore always belated—involves a flight from death, from the impossible possibility and possible impossibility.

As (im)possibility, however, death is possibility pure and simple, possibility that can never be actualized and to which nothing real ever corresponds. For this reason one cannot expect death. The possibility of the impossibility, that is possibility itself, never coincides with an attitude of expectation: "Expectation is not just an occasional looking away from the possible to its possible actualization but is essentially a *waiting for that actualization.* . . . In accordance with its essence [the possibility of the impossibility of existence] offers no support for becoming intent on something, 'picturing' to oneself the actuality which is possible, and so forgetting its possibility" (Heidegger [1], p. 307/262). The covering up of death, of its certainty and indefiniteness, turns out to be a covering up of the possibility that is the "ownmost possibility" of Dasein: only Dasein knows of the possibility itself. This knowledge does not correspond to holding as true a fact that can be experienced. Rather, it is the certainty of death as the "distinctive *certainty* of Dasein." Heidegger characterizes the ownmost and certain possibility of Dasein, the possibility of impossibility, possibility itself, which is not just one possibility among others, by emphasizing its indefiniteness: "the 'when' in which the utter impossibility of existence becomes possible remains constantly indefinite" (p. 310/265). Dasein is threatened "constantly" because it exists in the constant indefiniteness of the certainty of its death and must not "tone it down" [*abblenden*], but rather must "cultivate it" [*ausbilden*] if it wants to open itself up to its ownmost possibility. The constancy of Dasein, which must be distinguished from the "inconstancy" of "disconnectedness," from the "inconstancy" of a connectedness of life that is produced belatedly, is an opening onto the constant threat that lies in Dasein itself, in its condition of finitude. The threat is in no way external to Dasein just because it is not at its disposal, *and it could not be experienced at all without the constant indefiniteness of certainty.* The constancy and cultivation of this indefiniteness are inextricably linked. A Dasein whose existence is not defined by the indefiniteness of the certainty of its ownmost possibility is incapable of experiencing the threat. Thus it becomes evident that the tendency of certainty and definiteness to coincide, a tendency wherein looms the destruction of certainty, does not just threaten to close the opening onto the constant threat. It does not just pose a threat to the threat. It also modifies the effects of the anxiety that makes possible the "genuine disclosure" of this threat and the understanding of authentic Being-toward-death, because in the threat Dasein finds [*befindet*] itself "*facing* the 'nothing' of the possible impossibility of its existence" and because "all understanding is accompanied by a state-of-mind [*Befindlichkeit*]" (p. 310/265–66). Can Dasein then still be "itself"? Can "Being-a-whole" further reveal to Dasein its dispersion? Can Dasein "authentically understand" its "ownmost," "certain" possibility? Can Dasein "maintain itself in an authentic Being-toward-the-end," in a Being-toward-the-end that anticipates the ungraspable possibility of death, that discloses "all the possibilities which lie ahead of that possibility," thereby anticipating "the *whole* of Dasein"?

Against an interpretation that uses the emergence and epidemic spread of AIDS as the occasion to point out the consequences of turning the indefiniteness of the "when" into the definiteness of a point in time, one could raise two decisive objections. First, one could protest that such an interpretation misunderstands the indispensable dependency of the "when" on indefiniteness, that it conceives of the "when" only in terms of an everyday understanding of time, that is, in terms of the possibility of pinpointing a specific date. Would not the "when" remain indefinite even if one could calculate the year, the month, the day, even the hour of one's death? Does not AIDS expose us to a stronger certainty and thus to a greater indefiniteness? And does not AIDS accordingly provoke a flight from death into dispersion? One might also object to the interpretation in question by contending that it—not very differently from everyday Being-toward-death—downplays the possibility of dying at any moment: Is it not possible that a terminally ill person, who knows more or less when he will die, could meet with an unexpected, unpredictable accident that leads to a death "before his time," to a death that is "premature" with respect to the "prematurity" of the determinate death?

Any ability to pinpoint the specific date of the "when"—that is, to calculate the probability of a date of death—is insufficient to support the claim that indefiniteness (the necessary correlate of certainty) tends to turn into definiteness and in this way brings about the catastrophe of the totality of Dasein. As insufficient as that is, one must not neglect that talking about the "when" only makes sense if we somehow maintain the link through which the indefinite is always already assigned to a possible definability—to the definability provided by the time of a calendar, for instance. An absolutely indefinite "when," a "when" that has shed even the last trace of definability, would no longer be a "when." Even in situations where a "when" cannot be defined in terms of (present-at-hand) time, in situations where the indefinability of something that never falls into time must be assumed, the tension between indefinability and definability remains. And it remains independently of how one conceives of it and the degree of its resistance to *comprehension.*[14] Being-not-one with AIDS seems to cause this tension to be felt acutely. But how should the "immediacy" that induces Heidegger to speak of the radical indefiniteness of the "when" be understood, and how the "at-any-moment"? How is death—the "uttermost and authentic possibility" that Dasein anticipates in order to disclose a temporality arising from the future of this possibility, and in order to exist in its "authentic potentiality-for-being-a-whole"—how is death related to the "moment" of "authentic temporality" that maintains itself in resoluteness, frees Dasein from dispersion, and permits the disclosure of Dasein's actual "there"? Is dying a moment? Does one die in a moment?

It seems justified to insist on the fact that one could die at any moment and that even the definability of the "when" does not change anything. But it might be argued that indefiniteness, while not simply vanishing within the bewildering perspective opened up by such "definability," nevertheless undergoes a modification that must be taken into account. The experimental, clarifying, and as it were exaggerated delineation of this modification could be labeled as the tendency of certainty and definiteness to coincide.

What would it mean to exhibit a Being-not-one, which consists in the definiteness of certainty? What would it mean to exhibit it *as such*? Would the exhibition of Being-not-one *as such* not be (to employ a somewhat formulaic expression, but one meant to respond concisely to the challenge posed by the virus) a *Being-not-at-one in Being-not-one*?[15] Would it not be a Being-not-one and a Being-not-at-one (neither exists without the other) that no longer aim at Being-one, that no longer need to concede that they remain powerless and reactive because of the belatedness of the question that asks for a restitution of the connectedness of life? Would this not be a Being-not-at-one that does not simply perpetuate Being-not-one? Originary Being-not-one, originary not-belonging does not resist Being-one, identity, belonging; it does not compete with them and does not challenge them; it is not subject to the opposition between belonging and not-belonging, between identity and lack of identity, between Being-one and Being-not-one. The exhibition of Being-not-one as such is also not an understanding that institutes an (originary) totality, but an exposure without a whole. Perhaps one only has time to live and time to die when one is neither indebted to an identity nor reduced to its opposites, disruption and fragmentation. Perhaps one has this time—without having it at one's beck and call—in originary Being-not-one, in originary not-belonging, in originary im-pertinence.

Does Being-not-one with AIDS thereby become the legitimating *sign* of this originary im-pertinence, this originary Being-not-one, which cannot actually be labeled and legitimized? How one encounters AIDS is not decided by whether one justifies it, but by the way one does so.[16] *Either* one justifies Being-not-one by negating it and linking it back to the unity of time, the self, and the connectedness of life (in which case one gives oneself over to the reactive and stands in danger of immortalizing the anxiety or anger caused by dying "before one's time"), *or* Being-not-one is "justified" because Being-not-at-one measures up to it and so affirms it (in which case one may have a chance against the impotence of the reactive, the power of which, as is well known, is the power of *ressentiment*). It is unbearable and unimaginable that a person one loves is meant to die, that he is meant to die of the consequences of AIDS. One cannot and must not engage with the certainty of his (more or less) definite death. All words of consolation, of appeasement, and of explanation cannot and must not be endured; one cannot and must not be satisfied with all the well-meant measures taken and initiatives launched, with all the traditional and conventional thought patterns that in the final analysis justify AIDS because they do not measure up to it, responding to its challenge with unusable concepts, with concepts that are undoubtedly familiar and recognizable, but which regularly lull one into a false sense of security.

§ 2 The Epidemic as a Rupture in History

Thesis for a retrospective assessment: It will have been said about AIDS that something reaches its end with the spreading of the virus— for the time being or permanently.

The spread of AIDS is not seen simply as the appearance of a new disease that could be integrated into an already existing continuity, an order of things. It is perceived as a rupture, provoking urgent testimony and confession. Thinking and talking about the virus are defined to a large degree by attempts to acknowledge this rupture—and possibly also to reject or repress it. Certainly, it is a matter of a break with the ideas of modern medicine, which aims at "the end of all disease" (Bounan, p. 70), but even more so of a rupture within the individual and between the individual and others: Being-not-one with AIDS. At this point three general questions can be posed:

1. What are the relationships between a rhetoric of medical objectivity and the symbolic force that invests disease, especially AIDS, and feeds on scientific statements precisely because such statements are already preformed by rhetorical constructions of social reality? In fact, these constructions make it difficult to draw any distinction between material bases and ideological formations. In an essay on AIDS, Paula A. Treichler writes: "Science is not the true material base generating our merely symbolic superstructure.

27

Our social constructions of AIDS (in terms of global devastation, threat to civil rights, emblem of sex and death, the 'gay plague,' the postmodern condition, whatever) are based not upon objective, scientifically determined 'reality' but upon what we are told about this reality: that is, upon *prior* social constructions routinely produced within the discourses of biomedical science. (AIDS as infectious disease is one such construction.) . . . No clear line can be drawn between the facticity of scientific and nonscientific (mis-) conceptions" (Treichler [1], pp. 35 and 37).

   2. Why has AIDS been singled out more than any other severe affliction as the measure of the time in which we live? "We now have that metaphor: with its links to sex, drugs, blood, and informatics, and with the sophistication of its evolutions and of its strategy for spreading itself, AIDS expresses our era." This statement is a synopsis of the preface to the history of the AIDS epidemic written by the historian Mirko D. Grmek (p. xii/19). Donna Haraway's study on the "determinations of the self" in biopolitical discourse, specifically in discourse about the immune system, describes the understanding of disease prevalent today and addresses why AIDS circulates in our language and imaginations as a metaphor *for* the epoch and as a metaphor *of* the epoch: "Disease is a subspecies of information malfunction or communications pathology; disease is a process of misrecognition or transgression of the boundaries of a strategic assemblage called self. . . . Immune system discourse is about . . . [the] possibility for engaging in a world full of 'difference,' replete with non-self" (Haraway, pp. 15 and 18).

   3. One hypothesis about AIDS traces the rupturing effects that accompany the emergence and spread of the virus to the lack of an effective vaccine or a successful therapy, even to the circumstance that "none of the factors that cause AIDS are presently opposed" (Bounan, p. 125). Another hypothesis emphasizes the irreversible, unpreventable, indelible, and unique qualities of those interruptive effects. If we can say that talking about AIDS happens in a space limited by these two juxtaposed and mutually exclusive hypotheses, where should we stand, which position should we take? How relevant and revelatory is the time of AIDS? What is

the importance of the epoch that supposedly expresses AIDS, if we stand in a divided space, in a space not identical with itself? How should we represent or imagine AIDS?[1] Only this last question will be discussed at greater length and in more detail below.

If the emergence and epidemic spread of AIDS brings to conclusion a period of time, a relatively short period, which can be distinguished as a period, can be marked, recognized, and identified, then this period—or more precisely this epoch—would have to be called the epoch of tricks. But what is a trick?[2] What does Renaud Camus, who wrote the book *Tricks*, mean by his title? A *trick* is a "first encounter," an encounter that happens only once, that comes only once; in order for one to speak of a *trick*, however, "something must emerge"; in order for a *trick* to happen [*kommt*], there must be cum. If now a third element is added to these two elements of the definition, namely, the particularity of the encounter ("that which remains comparable in each encounter, but nevertheless doggedly asserts itself as something *specific* and *unique*"), one ascribes to the *trick* the quality of an experience. For any experience worthy of the name must comprise at least these elements: something must begin, something must happen, and something must remain comparably unique, unique while comparable. *Trick* is the name given to an experience of homosexuality. But if one assumes with Camus that "before having a . . . *nature*, homosexuality has a history," that it is "an *experience* before being an essence," one can ask what it is that befalls the experience and history of homosexuality called *trick*, during the epoch that is distinguished by the emergence and spread of AIDS.

Renaud Camus added prefatory remarks to the numerous editions and translations of his book, which was printed for the first time more than ten years ago. At this juncture, it might be worthwhile to focus on the preface to the German edition. It was written in 1986 and is characterized by confession and testimony, by the vindicating admission of a loss of innocence. "The plague and the passing of the years have given this book the character of a historical document: the world it describes is to a large extent a past world. There is no doubt that one has to relinquish this particular world—hopefully only for the time being. Applying absolutely necessary precautions, one must adapt to the new, calamitous situation. But I will not deny the nostalgic affection that I hold for this world, for its droll, carefree gaiety, its liveliness, its late nights and early morning hours, its innocence" (Camus, p. 25). What are the consequences of the rupture and the discontinuity that turn the previously innocent, light, carefree book into a "historical document" burdened with the spirit of gravity, infecting innocence and exposing it to (nostalgic) intention and hidden thoughts? In its transformation, in its historicity, the book from now on bears witness to an epoch,[3] since the very notion of a "historical document" is inseparably linked to the concept of the epoch, that is, to the concept of that which distinguishes itself as a more or less unique period within a more or less universal history. But if one interprets the rupture as such a transformation and historization, then one must understand it as a rationalization. One must understand it in terms of the recuperating justification that characterizes all testimony insofar as it testifies to something, to some determinate thing. History and experience become integrated into a meaningful whole: they become essence and nature.

Roland Barthes wrote a preface to *Tricks*. In it he claims that there is one thing "society will not tolerate," namely, that "I should be . . . *nothing*, or to be more exact, that the *something* that I am should be openly expressed as provisional, revocable, insignificant, inessential, in a word: impertinent." An existence that—going back to the etymology of the word—is *im-pertinent*,[4] an existence that does not let itself be determined and therefore claims no right to existence, would not only have to resist all attempts to circumscribe and delimit it, to pin it down; it would also have to be a limit that through its lack of discursive meaning makes discourses possible. It would have to be a limit from which one could introduce distinction into discourse and thus unfold a discourse. Doesn't Barthes already open the distinction itself to something that cannot be distinguished, that is neither positive nor negative, and without which there can be no distinctions, when he distinguishes those who find in the homosexuality of others a pretext for

showing off their liberal attitudes from those who testify as homosexuals to what they endure because of their identity, because of
an identity they ascribe to themselves and that is ascribed to them
by others?

If one wanted to describe more precisely the im-pertinent as the
limit of discourse, it would be necessary first to ask what a limit is
and how it is drawn. In this context, Kant's distinction between
limits [*Grenze*] and bounds [*Schranke*] turns out to be helpful. It is
a distinction used in the *Critique of Pure Reason*[5] and drawn again
in section 57 of the *Prolegomena*, where he opposes limits to
bounds. This section concludes the treatment of "the determination of the bounds of pure reason," and reproaches skepticism as
originating in the "unpoliced dialectic" of metaphysics. Do not the
police attempt to limit transgressions? While bounds are "mere
negations which affect a quantity as far as it is not absolutely complete," "in all limits there is something positive." Limits concern
extended beings and as such "presuppose a space existing outside a
certain definite place and inclosing it" (Kant [1], pp.
99–103/351–54). Limits, therefore, are meaningful only where extension and spatiality permit a division and a distribution. Their
positive aspect lies in the fact that they themselves are spatial or a
place in space, that they indicate another space, even if we recognize nothing in that space and can think the things that fill it only
with recourse to the limiting concept of a noumenal world. Kant
states: "But our reason, as it were, sees in its surroundings a space
for knowledge of things in themselves, though we can never have
definite concepts of them and are limited to appearances only" (p.
101/352).[6]

The difference between limit and bound, which results from the
fact that the former is essentially positive, whereas the latter is a
mere negation, appears as a difference within knowledge and seems
to take a hierarchical form. In the extensive infinity of its inner
progress, mathematical knowledge never reaches a limit because it
is not in need of morals or of metaphysics. Both morals and metaphysics lie outside mathematical knowledge, and as this outside
they form its bounds, bounds to which it does not relate.[7] But the

relative independence of mathematical knowledge, defined by bounds, depends in the final analysis on the unity of reason and on the unity of the system, the possibility of which is examined and established by the critical propaedeutics of metaphysics, that is, by a thought of the limit.

Bounds are not limits, because they distinguish the homogeneous rational knowledge of a "sphere" from that which remains foreign to this sphere and must remain im-pertinent with respect to it. Limits, in the Kantian sense, are drawn where heterogeneity occurs within a sphere, separating rational knowledge from itself, and only thus making it possible. Without the constitutive moment of heterogeneity, every limit would erase itself instantly. In contrast to the bound, the limit is a critical concept. And this concept must be considered inasmuch as the disconnectedly heterogeneous—the known and the entirely unknown—is connected and thus creates the possibility of a meaningful use of reason. According to this logic, one can maintain oneself on a limit but not on a bound. To the degree that limits not only keep things separate but also unite them, bring them together and link them, they are the expression of "a relation to something"; they indicate that the known presupposes the unknown and functions as the indication of that which is presupposed. (Kant uses the word *Anzeige* [indication] in the *Prolegomena*: in retrospect, his use can be read as announcing Wittgenstein's use of the word *Zeigen* [showing, indicating].)[8] For this reason it is possible to bring "into clarity" the "concept of the connection" that exists between the presupposed unknown and the indicating known. The produced clarity allows us to maintain ourselves on a limit. "But we maintain ourselves on this limit," Kant explains, "if we limit our judgment merely to the relation which the world may have to a Being whose very concept lies beyond all the knowledge which we can attain within the world. For we then do not attribute to the Supreme Being any of the properties in themselves, by which we represent objects of experience, and thereby avoid *dogmatic* anthropomorphism; but we attribute them to the relation of this Being to the world and allow ourselves a *symbolical* anthropomorphism, which in fact concerns language only and not the object itself" (Kant [1], pp. 105–6/357).

To sum up: a limit always distinguishes itself by a peculiar heterogeneity of the homogeneity of the sphere, which alone secures the ground for the production of a connection and a relation. If it is merely a question of a delimitation between two spheres which in themselves are homogeneous, then we are dealing not with a limit, but rather with a bound. At this point, however, the question could be posed whether the heterogeneity of the homogeneity of the sphere, which defines, distinguishes, and articulates the limit, must not always also be restrictive, in the negative sense of a bound as described by Kant. For heterogeneity is heterogeneous only if it also interrupts, if something in it remains without connection, without indicating function, without relation. This is perhaps the point where a distinction between limit and bound can no longer be stabilized, but all the more urgently requires stabilization. Paradoxically formulated: limits exist only insofar as they carry *in themselves* a de-limitation or restriction, which itself restricts the distinguishing identification. Kant remarks that statements about the heterogeneous relation that underlies all relations concern only language but not the object; he refers to statements about the relation of the unknown to the known, of the outside to the inside, of that which lies outside knowledge to that which is known within the world. Can he be understood as saying that the interruption of this relation, which is inextricably connected with its production and happens within it, gives us over to a language that threatens the unity of reason because, at a definite but never-determinate point, it ceases to be a discursive, distinguishing, and identifying, that is, a referential language?

In that case, it would not only be the confusion of bound and limit that is im-pertinent, but also the limit itself in its limiting and delimiting capacity, the limit as distinguished from the bound. Not only are limit and bound not-one, the limit is not-one in and with itself. Kant himself testifies to this Being-not-one, without which there is no limit and without which no unity, given that a unity can be thought only on the limit. On the one hand, he insists on the impossibility of experiencing an absolute limit. In his posthumous papers there is a note that distinguishes that which delimits from that which is delimited; limits as limits of phenomena (what has limits, if not phenomena?) are attributed to that which is limited: "The limit of the phenomenon is part of the phenomenon, but the thing that creates the limit is outside it. Therefore we have reason to assume a being that is the origin of the world and of a future world, but we have no means to determine this being" (Kant [3], p. 41 [Refl. 4958]). On the other hand, one has to distinguish the limits of phenomena from these phenomena; one has to delimit the limit in order to escape being caught in the infinite regression from the determined to the determined. There is always something in the (phenomenal) limit that is also an absolute limit. As stated in the *Prolegomena*, the "limit belongs to the field of experience as well as to that of intelligible beings" (Kant [1], pp. 105/356–57). The Being-not-one of the limit (a limit unites and interrupts) marks its difference from a simple bound. Thus, the Being-not-one creates a position from which to think a unity and render knowledge possible. But it also prevents the limit from being brought fully "into clarity"—it doesn't allow us to distinguish consistently between the limit and that which it delimits.

On such a limit, an im-pertinent limit meant to prevent impertinence, one cannot maintain oneself untroubled. No police are capable of making it entirely secure. If one wants to think impertinence—Being-not-one—not as the opposite of unity, belonging, and pertinence but as originary im-pertinence, one must describe it as a limit. The idea of an im-pertinent existence or an originary Being-not-one is essentially constituted by its being a limit that is always stabilized but never reaches stability. The (impassable) limit is originary im-pertinence; originary im-pertinence must be a limit. This essential constitution of originary im-pertinence as an unstable limit (ultimately a redundant formulation) leads us to think existence as exposure, as Being-expose prior to all positing. Existence is exposed as originary Being-not-one, as a limit, which cannot be distinguished without difficulty from a bound. But this does not mean that originary Being-not-one co-incides with death: existence is that which is implied in the most stable form of identity, even if such an identity can never recover, secure, stabilize, or identify it.

In order to establish the claim that the transformation of a re-port, a narration, a representational sequence into a "historical document" always overtakes and rationalizes existence, we want to rely on the idea of an originary im-pertinence, a primordial Being-not-one, a limit that in its essence is not secured; we want to refer to an existence that originally cannot be distinguished and differ-entiated. But can one rely on such an idea? Can one refer to such an existence? Such a transformation into a historical document oc-curs independently of any particular will or distinct intention. It is also possible, however, that the author intends and wants it. But stating after the fact that a narrative has become a "historical doc-ument" is not quite the same thing as wanting to write something that will become a "historical document." The American writer David Leavitt has declared on several occasions that one day he would like to read his own works and be able to say to himself, "If you want to learn something about the fight against AIDS, read David Leavitt" (*El País Semanal,* Jan. 28, 1990, p. 25).

The epidemic emergence of AIDS, as should have become clear by now, had the effect that (finite) existence, threatened by the virus, was integrated into a recognizable history and into a history of recognition, thus transcending its finitude. Of course, discourses practicing inclusion or inscription are often mutually incompatible and furthermore correspond to diverse or even opposite feelings and attitudes: they do not correspond to *one* consciousness. But the militant lament, the active mourning of a lost freedom, and its violent negation—negation also in the psychoanalytic sense of a denial—resemble each other inasmuch as they refer back to a fi-nite existence, the history of which makes sense and which thus sheds its finitude. Before taking on a precise, determinate, articu-lated meaning or sense, history already makes sense. It can be rec-ognized—the past or present representation of the historical can become a "historical document." That the epidemic emergence of

AIDS makes sense because it marks a historical rupture is confirmed by Susan Sontag's observation that the outbreak of the epidemic is perceived not as a natural catastrophe, a catastrophe of nature (at least not in the West), but as an event of history, a historical event. As it spreads across the West, the virus or the syndrome called AIDS becomes a historical phenomenon. Its status differs from that of the diseases that ravage the nations of the poorest continents. We know, for example, that speculative philosophy declares Africa to be a continent, a part of the world, that lacks history, a part of the world one can leave without recollecting or remembering it later. Africa is the "undeveloped land which is still enmeshed in the natural spirit"; it remains steeped in the night of a not yet awakened self-consciousness and forms but the limit the "threshold of world history" (Hegel [1b], p. 190/129).[9] This example, of course, is not just an example, because speculation wants to show that world history is the "unfolding" of the spirit in time and that this movement of the spirit is analogous to the movement in the course of which the idea "unfolds" as space in nature.[10] "Part of the self-definition of European and neo-European countries," Susan Sontag writes, "is that . . . the First World . . . is where major calamities are history-making, transformative, while in poor, African or Asian countries they are part of a cycle, and therefore something like an aspect of nature" (Sontag, 171–72).

Two reasons can be cited in order to justify recourse to the word "trick," trick as the name of an epoch before AIDS, a temporal unity that can be delimited and recognized from the viewpoint of a historical rupture. First, "trick" in the wider sense signifies the multiplication of singular and comparable encounters that involve sexual intercourse, regardless of their sexual specificity. It stands for that "liberalization of sexual . . . mores" that was no less meaningful than the return to monogamy, to an alleged stability, the valorization of which remains indissociable from the rapid, worldwide spread of the infection (cf. Grmek, p. 109/187). Second, a "trick," in the narrower sense of a homosexual encounter, makes the liberalization experienced in the 1960's and 1970's all the more obvious: the "trick" as the wide screen of the "sexual revolution."

Commenting on the number of homosexuals who once lived in certain areas of San Francisco, the historian Grmek notes that "never in human history had one city known such a concentration of homosexuals, nor such promiscuity." As questionable as is the comparison with the "whole history of humankind,"[11] it points to the epochal importance of its object: "The pursuit of physical pleasure and multiple partners passed for fundamental expressions of individual rights" (Grmek, pp. 169/276–77). From the point of view of a sociologist, Pollak notes that urban middle class homosexuals "turned the development of their sexuality into an ideal of life, at once the engine and result of a liberation movement claiming rights" (Pollak, pp. 28–29). What emerges from this schema, which allows us to speak of an "epoch" of the "trick," is that existence and the freedom ascribed to it are determined with respect to a (*historical*) *identity*. To the subject who seeks his identity in the sacralization of sexuality corresponds, after the historical rupture, a responsible subject after the historical break, that is to say, a subject who has "converted" to "new forms of sexuality." Hygienic care and self-control, the "desacralization," reflected in a "ritualization of safer sex" (Pollak, p. 81),[12] mark "the culmination of a long process of civilization that has given birth to the notions of rights, dignity, and respect" (p. 167).

Thus, the first coming out of homosexuals is doubled and, so to speak, outstripped by a second one. Now coming out consists of an integration by which the subject constitutes itself as a part of the "common cause" of those directly or indirectly affected by AIDS: the cause of the *AIDS community*.[13] In this context, one has to remember the struggle waged in the United States, and especially in New York, by the group *ACT UP*.[14] But integration into a common cause, a cause of a community, can also belong to a certain American ideology, as evidenced by films such as *Longtime Companion*. (How one relates to movies that, due to the circumstances of their production, serve ideological purposes, depends strongly on the general question of the political. For example, is one supposed to welcome the movie *Philadelphia* by Jonathan Demme [1993] simply for the reason that it is publicized as the first serious, large-scale treatment of AIDS in the Hollywood manner? Or should one pay attention to the film's recourse to conventional mechanisms of identification, to its minimizing of political contents, to its portrayal of the sexual as innocuous, to its obsessive fixation on sexuality, to the use of its topic for the celebration of a sense of justice that distinguishes, at least ideally, American society? Does this film blind the spectator?) We might say that AIDS encourages a "withdrawal into oneself," as well as social commitment and public witnessing (Pollak, pp. 106 and 116). If homosexuals, as the medical historian claims, provided "the ideal 'culture medium' in which, as though in a laboratory experiment, the virus could multiply during its critical phase" (Grmek, pp. 170/278–79), then their first *coming out* actually paved the way for the second by providing the conditions necessary for a sociological experiment. Sociology teaches us that the epidemic spread of AIDS created a "quasi-experimental situation" that put to the test the "values of tolerance and of individual freedom" and "the ability of modern society to react quickly to an unexpected threat" (Pollak, pp. 13–14).[15]

Certainly, it has already been understood that the construction of a (double) historical identity, which is guided by the assessment that a historical rupture has taken place, deprives itself of the very means of thinking that rupture, and in the same gesture conceals that which has even stronger effects than the rupture: the idea of an originally im-pertinent existence, a Being-not-one that is neither opposed to Being-one nor determined by it. It is not a matter of deciding whether the emergence and spread of AIDS have put an end to an epoch, whether we can recognize in the rupture a chance to create a new responsibility and a new identity. Nor is it a question of integrating oneself into a "quasi-experimental situation." Rather, it is a question of thinking what AIDS might mean for an existence without historical identity, for an existence that testifies to nothing and has nothing to confess. For such an existence, AIDS would have no meaning, not because it dispenses with protecting itself against the infection, not because it gives in to irresponsibility and indifference, admitting only the negative significations of defeatism, nihilism, and obscurantism, but because its im-pertinence consists in exposing distinguished and distinguishing, differentiated and differentiating meaning to that which cannot be differentiated, to the "*something* that I am." This "something" cannot be fixed by opposing it to something else; for every "something" is, as Hegel points out, another. Every deictic "this" that is supposed to distinguish something else or something other falls "outside the something" (Hegel [2], p. 117/126), as every proper name something bears can be "arbitrarily assumed, given, or also altered."

In *The Time of AIDS*, Michel Bounan maintains that precisely the system that engenders "the set of . . . factors" causing AIDS also "funds the research and directs the researchers" (Bounan, p. 125). But is it possible to measure the weight of such a claim if one opposes a "living whole" to the market, to a society of commodities and to the civilization within which such a society constitutes itself? Bounan reproduces the discriminations and determinations of such an existence by subscribing to a discourse that remains caught in opposites and is thus limited. In fact, it is difficult for the reader to distinguish the oppression within the social order analyzed by Bounan from certain repressive traits that mark his analysis of "the time of AIDS" as an age of "extreme servitude." Homosexuality seems to be completely identified with a "sexual perversion," whose social function depends on the "dominant class," and whose very origin and persistence coincide with the existence and permanence of different classes within society (p. 110).

But if the totalizing denunciation of "sexual freedom" moves in a space limited by oppositional discourse, if this discourse imposes its own limits on the gesture of denunciation, one should also mistrust those discourses that ascribe to "sexual freedom" the value of autonomy. These discourses assimilate sexual experience to the overcoming of violence and abolition of all discrimination. AIDS precludes no hyperbole. In his essay "Is the Rectum a Grave?," which appears in a collection on AIDS, Leo Bersani proclaims a new "celebration" of male homosexuality. With this polemical announcement he attempts to acknowledge and accept the "obsession" that supposedly characterizes the relationship of homosexuals to sexuality. Obsession brings to view the risk that Bersani situates in sexuality itself, "the risk of self-dismissal, of *losing sight* of the self" (Bersani, p. 222). This risk of sacrificing the self, however, is embedded in a movement that can make it disappear: "It is possible to think of the sexual as, precisely, moving between a hyperbolic sense of self and a loss of all consciousness of self. But sex as self-hyperbole is perhaps a repression of sex as self-abolition" (p. 218). The abolition, extermination, overcoming, or transgression made possible by sexuality and staged in the act demonstrate, according to Bersani, a practice of nonviolence (p. 222). Undoubtedly, the concept of nonviolence introduced by the author at the end of his essay requires further discussion—can the relinquishing of the self not also be a sanctioning of violence? But for our purposes it will suffice to point out that an essential relation exists between (homo-)sexual transgression or overcoming and (discriminating) differentiation. As soon as sexuality receives its definition from that which cannot be defined and which can *suppress* its own hyperbolic movement, as soon as homosexuality is accorded the privilege of bringing this definition of the indefinable to light and making it visible—homosexuality as a wide screen—one already differentiates and discriminates against that which does not permit any (discriminating) differentiation. One pushes experience into the neighborhood of essence. One attempts to subdue (originally im-pertinent) existence by means of a rationalization or recuperating justification.

In conclusion one could perhaps establish the following claim: those who proceed from the assumption that with the emergence and spread of AIDS something comes to a more or less abrupt, a more or less violent end, those who cite a historical rupture that permits them to distinguish two epochs, seem to erase precisely the very thing to which they wish to testify and for which they wish to give justification. AIDS renders (geopolitical, social, economic, national, cultural, ethnic, sexual) boundaries permeable and tears down the limits that have been established. For this reason only a thinking of primordially im-pertinent existence, of originary Being-not-one is capable of measuring up to the destructive force of the virus.

Sociological analyses indicate that many reactions triggered by the threat of AIDS can be traced back to precisely the im-pertinence that resists rationalization, recuperation, and any inference of a supporting ground. Are the implications of im-pertinence exhausted in its functioning merely as a reactive sign? "By causing fear of social rejection the expression 'risk group' first and foremost leads to a refusal: one refuses to let oneself be labeled. But this rejection of the stereotype is inscribed not only in a symbolic struggle, whose object is the defense of the public image of homosexuals. It brings to the fore the real fear of those who—unconcerned with their contradictory statements—feel exposed to a fatal risk and *who at the same time want to know everything and to understand nothing*" (Pollak, p. 83; my emphasis). To know everything and understand nothing:[16] perhaps we can confront AIDS, perhaps we can face AIDS only when we refuse *to decipher* and *to interpret* the im-pertinence that manifests itself in such reactions. That is, when we no longer interpret this im-pertinence as what it *also* is, as rejection, refusal and denial, as symbolic struggle, defense of social prestige and expression of real anxiety. A primordially im-pertinent existence, *infected before all contagion*, faces AIDS, looks AIDS in the face, a face it actually does not have. For this existence lets itself be shaken by the virus without having anything to confess, and therefore without having anything to defend.

§ 3 "I Am Out;
Therefore I Am"

In his political essay *Constat,* the French linguist Jean-Claude Milner maintains that today only disease and death are recognized as forms of politics. The physician or the dying person occupies the place of the revolutionary. AIDS, "carrier of the infinite in its darkest and least transparent shape," is "the mummy of '68" (Milner, p. 60) and represents the transformation of the formula that equates politics with ethics into one that equates ethics with disease—or ethics with death.

It is questionable, however, that one need be content with identifying the social function of AIDS with such a form of depoliticization, regardless of the degree to which it actually takes this form. Perhaps the equation of ethics with disease is not just a depoliticizing, disintegrating substitute for the unity allegedly constituted by politics and ethics; perhaps AIDS also creates a space for revolutionary action, thereby mirroring a shift that takes place in the political sphere itself. Such a shift happens when the aggressor weakens the defenses from the inside, instead of harrying the exterior. This is the case with the (projective?) threat of minorities and refugees, which has at least a formal connection with the threat the virus represents, as Gilles Deleuze points out (Deleuze, p. 292). That a person directly afflicted by AIDS can be seen as the messenger of an order that overthrows the existing one, and consequently as a particularly heroic figure facing up to the deadly threat, becomes apparent when one reads an article from 1985 by Didier Gille and Isabelle Stengers. But is it possible to say that a person ill with AIDS faces up to the threat heroically, that he challenges death more or less consciously, and that for this reason he stands out from the crowd? In Gille and Stengers's article one finds the well-known identification of homosexual promiscuity with an experimental praxis and situation. The sexual behavior of a certain quantitatively meaningful group of homosexuals creates the conditions for conducting an experiment, one that is supposed to include them as participants. Those homosexuals who participated in an experimental praxis, who lived in an experimental situation, and whose example had to become relevant for AIDS research—for research of a sociological or medical-historical kind—were transformed into an outpost, a vanguard, a company of messengers or scouts who, sent ahead, are now in a position to report about a general threat, a threat unknown until now. Thus, by reporting, they can sound the alarm. From an objective point of view they are among the first who exposed themselves to the threat, knowingly or unknowingly. (But must not a hero always face up to death knowingly, consciously, and resolutely?) Their advance into dangerous territory—not only into the other order but also into the Other of order—affected and affects them directly.[1]

Gille and Stengers assume that to every new vaccine or antibiotic invented by humans there corresponds the emergence, or even the invention, of a new virulent agent, which turns out to be resistant to the defensive measures used against it. From this assumption one could conclude that there is neither defense nor attack—if one understands these as clearly distinguishable units—but only an open system of differential entries and functions. As such they are nothing other than the provisional markings of resistance—of resistance against resistance—split and therefore already marked in themselves. This system, which makes homosexuals visible to the degree that they are, at first, particularly afflicted by AIDS and so appear as a vanguard, the authors call "life itself." The exchange of bodily fluids, without which the AIDS epidemic would be unthinkable, and which constitutes one of the last uncontrolled interrelations between "nature" and "culture," is dangerous. It is dangerous exactly "like life itself, which does not move in a closed circle" (Gille and Stengers, p. 81).

The homosexual becomes a hero because, as a member of the vanguard, he exposes his body to a danger that has the name of life—of "life itself." It is clear, however, that this heroism must distinguish itself from the heroism characterized by a courageous giving up of oneself and selfless sacrifice. For the life and death of the AIDS-hero do not serve as a prototype [*Vor-bild*]. The forward position of the vanguard is meant to resist the political, psychological, aesthetic purposes of representation and identification. After all, how could the AIDS hero, the hero of "life itself," become a prototype? The hero of "life itself" becomes a prototype only to the degree that he is a defined hero, a homosexual, for example, who invokes his homosexual identity. "Life itself" is nothing that in its particularity could put forth universal claims of validity, as does a nation, a religion, or a conviction. For this reason, Gille and Stengers also speak of an "abstract, faceless idea." Out of passion, in search of experiences that arouse desire, AIDS-heroes, heroes who in the time of AIDS continue to write the history of heroic exploration of "life itself," explore the capacities of the body. They explore "in their own flesh what a body is, what it can do, and what it cannot bear. They tell us what we are, they remind us [today] that we are generators and users of bodily fluids" (p. 82).

Let us retain the following conclusion: if the hero in the time of AIDS does not prove himself in the name of a universalized particularity, if he cannot become a prototypical model because he does not represent anything and because he cannot be represented, if he acts only in the name of an "abstract, faceless idea," an idea that does not grant a face and that is nothing but that "something" Gille and Stengers do not want to circumscribe specifically,[2] then this hero does not actually exist. Even the idea of a heroic sacrifice offered to humankind participates in the model of a universalized particularity and of representation, for it necessarily contains the representation of a progress and an aim. The hero of "life itself" does not exist; he demands infinite recognition since he can never be recognized. His uniqueness derives from the fact that "life itself," the "something" that at bottom is neither mere nature nor the opposed culture that mediates it, always surpasses him so that he can neither act *in the name* of the "something" nor as a hero *of* the "something."[3] Only the forerunner and messenger who does not touch on anything that could be recognized and assimilated, and who therefore must remain unrecognizable himself, encounters the "something." Therefore it is not decisive, in the final analysis, whether the hero exposes himself to the threat knowingly or not, whether he recognizes the threat as such only after the fact, or whether he attempts to readjust his actions in light of it. For this threat endangers every form of knowledge meant to serve as an instrument of control. The "something" that is perceived as a threat permits only a recognition that must itself remain insufficient, because unrecognizability is the mark of the forerunner and messenger who has encountered it. It contains no potentiality of recognizable meaning. The message does not mediate the meaning of "life itself"; it does not grant the "something" a recognizable definiteness; it does not permit us to recognize the "something" as determinate. Rather, the "something" is the structure of the vanguard [*Vor-hut*], the outpost [*Vor-postens*], the forerunner [*Vor-boten*], the running-ahead-of-oneself [*Sich-selber-Vorausgehens*]; it is the structure and the movement of Being-not-one.

If AIDS, if the unheroic AIDS-hero, or the hero in the time of AIDS, explores this Being-not-one, if because of this exploration we thus face the task of an exposure of Being-not-one *as such*, then it can only be a matter, to speak with Wittgenstein, of transforming the problematic background of life into a sort of halo. It can only be a matter of leading a right life by not trying to dissolve or reduce to a preceding unity what is unsolved and insoluble. We have to affirm the irreducible Being-not-one of life *while transforming it*. From such a perspective, from the perspective of an affirming transformation, which is not just an additional perspective, AIDS is less the "mummy of '68" than an exploration that could effect a radical political upheaval, an upheaval of all institutions based on identity and identification. Being-not-at-one with AIDS is the "destructive character" in politics: "I am out; therefore I am."

If one recalls Nietzsche's attempt to think the aporetic relation of sickness and health, it becomes obvious how untenable, how nihilistic in its idealism, is a position that finds in Being-not-one with AIDS merely a negativity, a negativity that can itself become productive when it is put to work as a restituting confession. In the *Genealogy of Morals*, Nietzsche states that life is not just measured by the degree to which health is spared from sickness.[4] The less life is prone to sickness, the more it is sickened by its health. Nothing is as healthy and conducive of life as being sick. Precisely for this reason, the health of life is in need of "agents who make sick" [*Krankmacher*]. That the passage in question is concerned with the soul hardly changes anything in the shape of the argument. Again, an experimental behavior—a sort of animal experiment incomparable to any other animal experiment—decides what our relationship to life is and what attitude we take toward ourselves: "Our attitude toward *ourselves* is *hubris*, for we experiment with ourselves in a way we would never permit ourselves to experiment with animals. Carried away by curiosity we cheerfully vivisect our souls: what is the 'salvation' of the soul to us today? Afterward we cure ourselves: sickness is instructive, we have no doubt of that, even more instructive than health—*those who make sick* [*Krankmacher*] seem even more necessary to us today than any medicine men or 'saviors.' We violate ourselves nowadays, no doubt of it, we nutcrackers of the soul, ever questioning and questionable, as if life were nothing but cracking nuts; and thus we are bound to grow day-by-day more questionable, *worthier* of asking questions; perhaps also worthier—of living?" (Nietzsche [2], pp. 113/357–58) "Sickliness" [*Krankhaftigkeit*] is a condition of life that cannot be canceled, because it alone makes the human into that which he is, and which can never be determined or fixed. This capacity of being sick promises him the future that defines him as a forerunner and precursor, exposed to all determinations and fixations, and thus never absorbed in them, a suspending and enabling limit, im-pertinent and interrupted: "Man is more sick, uncertain, changeable, indeterminate than any other animal, there is no doubt of that. He is *the* sick animal: how has that come about? Certainly he has also dared more, done more new things, braved more and challenged fate more than all the other animals put together: he, the great experimenter with himself, discontented and insatiable, wrestling with animals, nature, and gods for ultimate dominion—he, still unvanquished, eternally directed toward the future, whose own restless energies never leave him in peace, so that his future digs like a spur into the flesh of every present—how should such a courageous and richly endowed animal not also be the most imperiled, the most chronically and profoundly sick of all sick animals?" (p. 121/367).

The relation between sickness and health is aporetic because sickness as the condition of health at the same time endangers health and can be its destruction. Thus, it can never be finally decided whether experimenting and exposing oneself strengthen or weaken life. On the one hand, the No said to life that results from displeasure with the aporia of one's own existence, and belongs in fact to this aporia, "brings to light, as if by magic, an abundance of tender Yesses" (Nietzsche [2], pp. 121–22/367–68). On the other hand, however, the "sick"—those who are broken by their very own condition—"are man's great danger": "the sick represent the greatest danger for the healthy; it is *not* the strongest but the weakest who spell disaster for the strong" (121f; *367f*).[5] The *political* danger of this text, of this thinking of an unavoidable and irreducible aporia (an aporia beyond which one can go or which one can avoid only if one negates life and arrests its forerunning movement) derives from the violent cancellation of the aporetic itself—which is aporetic only at the price of *precisely this danger.* It arises whenever one cannot tolerate the impediment to passage posed by the aporetic. The proposal of a French right-winger, for instance, that suggests the internment of people with AIDS in a so-called *sidatorium* and aims at establishing protective and impermeable boundaries between the healthy and the sick cannot be considered to be simply the prolongation of the complex thought process in the course of which Nietzsche recommends the separation of the sick from the healthy. How could one decide *in advance* or even *in retrospect* whether being sick is a monitory lesson that allows humans to live (on) and that determines their health, at least if their health is to be an affirmation and not a negation, or whether being sick becomes a "warning" for the healthy, the "embodied reproach" that negates life and health? To pose the question differently, namely in relation to contemporary experiences of being sick: How can one make a conclusive and unequivocal proposition about Being-not-one with AIDS that fixes its meaning? Being-not-one forces us to be not-one and to be not-at-one. The irreducibility of Being-not-one, the necessity of exhibiting it *as such*, the powerlessness, futility, reactivity, and inertia of all attempts to refer it back to a Being-one are inscribed in it as the strangely shapeless shape of this Being-not-one, this fundamental undecidability, that always already affects its possible meaning.

Milner's assessment may be supported and even motivated by the fact that AIDS policy in the United States revived political activism. At the same time, perhaps because the effects of activism cannot be easily anticipated, its revival demonstrates how difficult it is to identify AIDS as "the mummy of '68." The way that leads to that mummy, and that supposedly makes Milner's identifying diagnosis possible, is a labyrinthine one. Or does the power of Milner's assessment depend precisely on finding shortcuts and tearing down walls? In that case, the labyrinthine nature of the way matters little for an assessment that opens the perspectives of thinking and life only because the assessment is itself a mummifying agent. Activism, the consciousness of the necessity and even the primacy of political action, seems to revolve around the problem of identity, at least in its dominant form, that is the form of gay activism. Its question is: How can we be one with AIDS? This question, by means of which gay activism sets off the depoliticizing effects to which Milner refers, can be divided into several different questions. There is the question of the *who*, concerning the addressees of thinking and talking about AIDS. There is the question of the *what*, concerning what happens in thinking and talking about AIDS. And finally there is the question of the *how*, concerning the possibility of thinking and talking about AIDS at all. Of course, these questions become meaningful only because they emerge from practical political experience and because they are directed toward making powerful and effective action possible. Thinking and talking about AIDS cannot be detached from the context of practical politics; they are inscribed in it and create it with the first word and the first thought. It is not possible here to discuss in depth whether thinking and talking about AIDS can be one with action and political practice, whether discourse and action, theory and practice, can and should pass into one another seamlessly, or whether their unfolding depends, rather, on a discontinuity,[6] which if crossed out turns action and practice into a pseudo-activity.

Who thinks—with whom and for whom—about AIDS? Who talks—with whom and for whom—about AIDS?

Douglas Crimp, in an instructive interview with Cathy Caruth and Thomas Keenan entitled *The Aids Crisis Is Not Over*, leaves no doubt that one cannot just think and talk about AIDS without asking the question of whom it is one addresses. To whom does Crimp address himself in the moment he denounces the fiction of a general public, of a homogeneous circle of addressees? To which public does this critique of ideology pave the way? Through critical reflection, we can already recognize what always turns out to be problematic in practice: "The biggest problem with even thinking about audiences is that one usually begins with some completely absurd fiction of generality, that is, with the notion that there could be a language that could reach everyone, or anything like a general public that could simply be addressed without exclusions. I don't think you could ever make any kind of cultural work that functioned as a general address. But the problem, of course, is that we live in a culture in which it is assumed that you can, always. And in fact almost every cultural work is made with that fiction of a general audience in mind" (Caruth and Keenan, p.

545). This discourse, which criticizes and exposes ideology, which reveals the concept of a general public to be a fiction of cultural work and of the culture in which this work is carried out, makes visible a structure of power and difference where differences and structures of power are supposed to have faded into the universality of equally distributed power. This is a discourse that chastises ideology in the name of concealed difference and imagines generality as always partial, intermittent, and particular, as always dependent on the acknowledgment of irreducible differences. Such a motivation, however, the motivation to denounce a fiction or an ideology in order to raise the question of AIDS properly, can also be presented programmatically; the intention of the discourse can become its explicit goal.

Thus a talk about *mourning* and *militancy*, published by Crimp in 1989, begins by emphasizing intention and gesture—as if the author wanted to say that no listener and no reader should doubt his goodwill, credibility, and honesty precisely because he does not address everybody, that is, because he cancels the ideological fiction of a general public of equal listeners and readers. This is a discourse of affliction setting the affliction into an immediate relationship with the fact of being concerned, of being affected by AIDS; it is a discourse of double identification: *of* and *with* addressees. Through this double identification, the discourse seems to exclude other identifications, but at the same time, its gesture of awareness of its own exclusivity, its self-reference as it were, has the unavoidable consequence that it must be understood just as much as an appeal for a general identification. This is a discourse of Being-one before and in the face of Being-not-one; it follows the general law that because I can identify (myself), I can address myself to, and talk to somebody else. Crimp addresses himself to his listeners and readers with these introductory remarks: "I, too, will have something to say about the distinction between self and not-self, about the confusion of the inside and the outside, but I am impelled to do this *for us*, for my community of AIDS activists. Writing about mourning and militancy is for me both necessary and difficult, for I have seen that mourning troubles us; by 'us' I

mean gay men confronting AIDS. It should go without saying that
it is not only gay men who confront AIDS, but because we face
specific and often unique difficulties, and because I have some familiarity with them, I address them here exclusively.[7] This paper is
written for my fellow activists and friends, who have also informed
it with their actions, their suggestions and encouragement—and
in this I include many women as well. The conflicts I address are
also my own, which might account for certain of the paper's shortcomings" (Crimp, p. 4). On the one hand, both the possibility of
a deconstruction of the notion of a public sphere that operates as a
critique of ideology and the possibility of an exclusive addressing-
oneself-to (the exclusive character of the address becomes intelligible only if it is linked to the deconstructive strategy) depend on
familiarity with the conflicts to which gay men confronted with
AIDS expose themselves. But on the other hand, it is precisely the
exclusive and excluding familiarity that causes a feeling of inadequacy, the feeling that the paper might be marked by some shortcomings. A negative dialectic is at work in this discourse: familiarity increases the strangeness of the familiar. This negative dialectic
is caused by the discrimination and the exclusion that make the
exclusive discourse possible and at the same time afflict it with inadequacy. How can one resolve conflicts, how can one do away
with the defects, the inadequacies, or the shortcomings of a speech
when this speech itself produces them? If it produces them, if it
does not just succumb to them, it is because of the structure of the
address that it vindicates as the only proper address, the only address it can justify. Are not the (activist) dream of a collective private language and the justified and justifying exclusivity of the address already compromised by the fact that the activist is capable of
identifying and naming the possibility of shortcomings? Why is
activism content with a deconstruction of the notion of a public
sphere that remains informed by a critique of ideology and that
replaces the ideological form of the general public with the transparent, unified, true medium of a particular public? Is activism incapable of bearing the differences it would like to advocate? Is it
intertwined with the concept of the public to such an extent that

the unrestricted, and not merely critical, deconstruction of this concept must also extend to activism itself? Is there activism without a (general or particular) public?

It is notable that the political problem of address, the problem of discursive practice—of addressing-oneself-to, of the addressee—turns out to be particularly urgent precisely in contexts affected by AIDS and AIDS policy, where one must ask how to relate to the emergence, spread, and politicization of the virus. The need to assert an identity, the need for a Being-one that integrates individuals, increases in the degree to which the identity of an individual, detached connectedness of life cannot be secured without being embedded in the unity of a more comprehensive connectedness. This need increases all the more when survival is linked to the force that allows the activist to assert Being-not-at-one and turn it into transforming practice. The activist is not-at-one with another identity or unity; the subject of activism is not-at-one with the subject of the state and the scientific institutions that conduct AIDS policy. If now this Being-not-at-one extends to the address itself, to its value-neutral universality—or more precisely, if this Being-not-at-one can only assert itself practically and politically as a Being-not-at-one with the ideological form of the general address, of an excluding inclusiveness—then the construction of a definite, separate (group) identity—and the limited, collective Being-one that guarantees this construction—must provide the possibility of a non-ideological address, an undisguised addressing-oneself-to-an-addressee. On what, however, could the identity and Being-one of homosexuals rely, the Being-one of homosexuals who are afflicted by AIDS? It is not a sufficient answer to say that one is stricken with the infection—even if in a quantitatively or qualitatively specific way. For in this case it cannot be clear enough how to draw the line of demarcation. The address marked out by this line contains two contradictory and therefore complementary dangers: the danger of restoring the fiction or ideology of universality—at least virtually everyone is affected by AIDS—and the danger of identifying AIDS with homosexuality. One reduces identity to a state of health, thus denying it;[8] or one affirms a reduced identity and makes it responsible for the disease, for the epidemic in general. Either case serves the veiled purposes of ideology or fiction.

In order to find a way out of the dilemma that is essential for activism—for gay activism—those for whom the political practice of Being-not-at-one is dependent on the possibility of tracing back Being-not-one to a Being-one often invoke the idea of a homosexual identity. They invoke an identity whose distinguishing feature is not AIDS and therefore does not exhaust itself in the subject's infection. The idea of such an identity assumes the shape or the defined form of an ideal. According to Crimp, what is mourned in the time of AIDS is "our ideal," that is, the ideal of a sexuality that distinguishes homosexuals from others and is supposed to grant them an identity, the ideal of a "perverse sexual pleasure" (Crimp, p. 11) that does not result from sublimation and only is what it is because it resists sublimation. The unspoken consequence of such a creation of identity and such mourning is that its instituting concept, the non-sublimated sexuality that is elevated as an ideal, is lost for a second time in mourning. This is the case at least insofar as the work of mourning can be associated with sublimation.[9] Mourning then becomes impossible or endless mourning, independent of AIDS and its effects. This is not to say, of course, that wherever AIDS leads to posing the question of mourning, the epidemic cannot be seen as a "wide screen" on which the necessity of a paradoxical, permanent mourning is projected. Does not the creation of an ideal itself already demand a sublimation, so that the loss of that which is elevated as an ideal— here, non-sublimated desire—and impossible, endless mourning are inscribed in the creation of the ideal? "Thus, the difficulty of mourning is certainly not gay men's alone. I only wish to emphasize its exacerbation for gay men to the extent that we are directly and immediately implicated in the particular cause of these deaths, and implicated, as well, through the specific nature of our deepest pleasures in life—our gay sexuality" (Crimp, p. 9*m*8). A homosexual identity oriented to the ideal of a definite sexuality, a definite sexual behavior, and for this reason a *homosexual* identity—

can there be another identity of those who identify themselves as homosexual?—does not exhaust itself, it is true, in being affected [Be*troffensein*] by the infection. But it is struck [ge*troffen*] in its essence by AIDS. In other words, when fighting the politics of the state, when attacking the indifference with which the suffering and dying of the ill is met, when denouncing the social stigmatization of the infected, the activist cannot avoid the dangers of an identification, of an equation of AIDS and homosexuality that creates identity, by having recourse to a sexual ideal that has already been mourned.

Sexuality can create collective and individual identity only when one ascribes a meaning to it, when one believes that it is possible to discover a meaning in it that exceeds any scientific, behavioral description. In his essay *The Ethics of Authenticity*, Charles Taylor points out that a "horizon"—the term originates in phenomenological hermeneutic philosophy—is necessary for the creation of identity. Only within the framework and environment created by a horizon can something become meaningful and contribute to self-definition. The solipsistic ascription of meaning and the arbitrary affirmation that the arbitrary is meaningful fail to recognize that an ideal collapses whenever it is not placed within a comprehensive horizon, which alone assigns it its meaning. The difference between a group and an individual becomes meaningful and creates an identity by placing itself in a shared horizon or, more precisely, in a horizon that encompasses individual differences and different identities. The negation of such a horizon, in which the ideal can endure—and it can endure only if it does so independently of our particular assignation of meaning—is, according to Taylor, the sign of nihilism.[10] "There is a certain discourse of justification of non-standard sexual orientations. People want to argue that heterosexual monogamy is not the only way to achieve sexual fulfillment, that those who are inclined to homosexual relations, for instance, shouldn't feel themselves embarked on a lesser, less worthy path." Taylor does not unfold all stages of the argument he outlines here. Homosexual tendencies are not just put side by side with heterosexual tendencies but are juxtaposed with "heterosexual monogamy." The symptomatic argument, of which Taylor gives a synopsis, thus implies a certain identification of promiscuity and homosexuality, *at least in the way it is presented by Taylor*; this identification, then, is relevant enough to distinguish homosexuals from heterosexuals. "This fits well into the modern understanding of authenticity, with its notion of difference, originality, of the acceptance of diversity. . . . Asserting the value of a homosexual orientation has to be done . . . empirically . . . taking into account the actual nature of homo- and heterosexual experience and life. It can't just be assumed a priori, on the grounds that anything we choose is all right" (Taylor, pp. 37–38). But how can the empirical orientation suggested by Taylor ever arrive at a meaning that stands within a "pre-existing horizon of significance," a horizon in which, for instance, the ideal of homosexuality, which creates identity, secures its continued existence as a recognized expression of difference?

The empirical investigation of homo- and heterosexual experiences cannot arrive at meaning itself, but at best at that which one might perceive as the expression, the impression, the reflection, or the tinge of meaning. However, is it thinkable at all that in the course of an empirical investigation one will uncover experiences or forms of life that can be identified by empirical means as "homosexual" and "heterosexual"? What exactly does Taylor designate as empirical reality or experience? How does the empirical relate to the horizon of meaning and significance that all empirical experience presupposes and is supposed to presuppose? Collective agreement, the production of which must already appear extremely problematic, no more guarantees the meaning of meaning than individual choice is a sufficient determinate of that which expresses itself as experience—that which experience itself ostensibly expresses. Collective agreement must articulate itself both in a group-specific agreement and in a comprehensive agreement that includes all specific groups. That is, it must articulate itself both in an agreement and in a unified and unifying agreement with the agreement. But such collective agreement cannot in itself cover the traces of the arbitrary, which condemns the decisionism of merely individual choice to powerlessness. The ambiguity of the concept of a pre-existing horizon, of a horizon that must constitute the vanishing point in any perspective, consists in the fact that this prefix can never turn itself into a positive ground just because agreement has been reached. Meaning instituted or established in order to make identity and difference possible, and to hold them together as such must also always transcend its establishment or institution. It must also always be a given meaning, a meaning instituted in a double sense, as, for example, the *Oldest System Program* stipulates.[11] Within the framework of a project that aims at the institution of such meaning, the task can only be to determine the relationship of the two institutions of meaning in that project: a purely created meaning (instituted from "inside") and a purely given meaning (instituted from "outside") coincide in an identity that has erased or sublated all differences. The purely created meaning is the purely given as pure identity, as indifference of meaning and meaninglessness. Therefore, difference means: the difference between creation and givenness, between two institutions (of meaning); it means the split of the institution itself, which does not permit a pure institution. Whereas absolute contingency and absolute necessity are one in the identity of pure creation and pure givenness, difference is the Being-not-one of the institution of a meaning that is always marked by a contingent, violent, arbitrary, conventional trait. There is meaning only in a Being-not-one that can never be reduced to meaning and never be put into a uniform, clearly defined, pre-existing, inescapable horizon of significance, although, to be sure, precisely this Being-not-one makes significance possible. This Being-not-one, if one may say so, is not-one with itself, and is never itself; it is never a *Being*-not-one and never has the uniform, identifiable meaning of *a* Being-not-one.

Precisely the difficulties that result for the *meaningful* creation of identity—and for a politics that depends on the recognition of identity—are mirrored in attempts to solidify the identity of the individual homosexual or of homosexuals through the establishment of a sexual ideal. The contingency, uncertainty, and uncontrollability of meaning, which themselves are constitutive of meaning,[12] can have dramatic consequences as the emergence and spread of AIDS shows. How is one supposed to control the meaning of the sexual ideal in the time of AIDS? In this context it is relevant that those who exalt the ideal of homosexuality are forced to defend contradictory and incomparable positions. In his book, *Policing Desire: Pornography, AIDS, and the Media,* Simon Watney, a British author particularly appreciated by North American activists, starts from an idealization of homosexuality that assigns homosexuality a privileged and exemplary meaning suitable for the establishment of identity. Watney then proceeds to the demand that this sexuality be curtailed. This demand concedes the loss of the sexual ideal and the connected, meaning-creating identity precisely by having to endow the curtailment of sexuality with new thrills and to proclaim this restriction as the source of new sexual *fantasies.* Although "it remains far from clear" that gay men and moralists have the same referent in mind when they talk about sex, Watney himself makes this difference evaporate. The heightening of *all* "erotic possibilities of the body" (Watney [1], p. 127) and its environment is meant to associate gay sex with the forbidden polymorphous perversity of the child. It is meant to distinguish gay sex from other forms of sexuality and thus invest it with a particular-universal meaning. Meaning is not immediately generated by sexuality; rather, it is generated by the interpretation of sexuality, by an implicit philosopheme, by the belief that sexuality *itself* is perceived in the practice of homosexuality beyond all exclusions and all systems of domination and oppression. Watney speaks of the strength of a "gay culture" that has helped homosexuals to their sexuality (ibid.). Wherever sexuality becomes an identity-creating sexual ideal, wherever it has a meaning and is meant to be sexuality *itself,* sexuality in its unadulterated, "natural" essence, it creates a culture and is no longer just "natural." But the instant that sexuality, which can assume all shapes and for that reason is sexuality *itself,* must be restricted and *should* be restricted[13]—this is a voluntary, suggested, recommended restriction, possible only because nature and culture are not in opposition here[14]—homosexual identity and meaning experience a crisis. In light of this crisis, it becomes considerably more questionable whether gay men, when talking about sex, can still identify the particularity of their referent and can thus distinguish themselves from other men.

In their study "Riding the Tiger: AIDS and the Gay Community," Robert A. Padgug and Gerald M. Oppenheimer transform the crisis of meaning as crisis of an identity guaranteed by a sexual ideal into a historical moment, a moment in the history of that which they designate as the "gay community." This history reaches its positive pinnacle with the creation of a "gay collectivity," which provides the fundament for "gay subjectivity." The authors do not hesitate to use expressions such as "truly 'homosexual'" (Padgug and Oppenheimer, p. 247). That they deal with the notion of homosexuality carefully, putting the adjective between quotation marks, does not prevent them from claiming in another passage, without quotation marks, that AIDS can never be "truly gay": "The disease had become gay in the circumstances of a specific historical conjunction, not because it was gay in any innate sense" (p. 258).

With the emergence and pandemic spread of AIDS, the second, negative pinnacle in the history of the "gay community" is attained and can receive a name. Because the authors assume a subjective and a collective historical identity, because they assume a historically gained autonomy and recognition, because they assume a historical becoming-visible and becoming-heard, because they assume the production of an identifiable public, in short: because they assume achievements that are also the conditions of address—of addressing-oneself-to—they can distinguish the world of gays from "the outside world" (p. 260). They can ask themselves how AIDS affected the community and what effects the community had on AIDS. And most of all they can pose the question of how the community may "control the social meaning of the disease" (p. 256). "*I am out; therefore I am*" means here: "I assume a fighting stance toward the outside because first and foremost I am at home in an inside."

If at a given historical point before the emergence of AIDS the

meaning of the "gay community" had already changed, if a movement concerned primarily with civil rights, which fought for
equality, tolerance, and institutional recognition, followed a political movement that aimed primarily at liberation from social repression, then one must not underestimate the crisis brought by
AIDS to the communally shared meaning. This crisis is not just
another moment in the history of the community, which could be
adopted and integrated by it. For the meanings linked to the liberation and civil rights movements are not sufficiently distinctive
and selective to work as criteria for the establishment of a "gay
identity," a "subjectivity" and a "community" of gay men.[15]

Again, the sexual ideal has to be invoked. But Padgug and Oppenheimer are anything but unequivocal when it comes to such
an ideal. The activities and institutions concerned with sexuality
are allegedly only one element of the "gay community"—even if
a special meaning adheres to this element. It seems that sexuality is
not affected by AIDS, at least not as such, not in its very essence or
nature. Padgug and Oppenheimer state that the spread of the
virus, which reaches epidemic proportions, leads to the abandonment of "particular *forms* of sexual expression . . . rather than gay
sexuality itself" (p. 261). However, that only a stronger "identification" with AIDS makes possible the control of its social meaning, that the effect of the epidemic on society consists of an assimilation of "gay sexuality" to other "forms of sexual expression," that
the readiness of gays and lesbians for a common fight against
AIDS and for cooperative solidarity announces the "decline of sexuality as a major component of gay identity" (p. 263)—these are
observations and claims indicating that without a sexual ideal that
is stable and beyond the reach of crisis the history of the gay community is in danger of losing its unity. The authors vacillate between two poles: they continually have to be repelled from one
and allow themselves to be attracted by the other, but neither the
sexual ideal nor the fight against the epidemic can save the truth of
gays and the identity-creating meaning of the word "gay." A history incapable of subsuming its critical moments under a meaning, a history whose meaning is not stabilized by the overcoming

of crises, is not a unified and continuous history any more, pervaded and supported by meaning. It is not a history of a community that is identical with itself and recognizes itself; it is not a common history that defines and determines its own identity. The control of meaning—which can, for example, assume the shape of either a reactionary or a progressive "policing of desire," which is either fought or supported by activism—is the condition for the constitution of historical identity.

Because uncontrollability and im-pertinence belong to meaning essentially, because they belong to the meaning of identity and identification[16] without ever being a part of meaning, attempts at exclusive and excluding address are bound to fail; any address that exclusively addresses a more or less homogeneous group, recognizable in its identity, and thereby attempts to exclude other identifiable groups, must fail because other meanings cannot be definitively excluded (for example, a different meaning ascribed to AIDS and its consequences by one outside the ostensible circuit of addressor and addressee). When Crimp addresses himself exclusively to his activist friends, when he emphasizes this exclusivity and thus makes clear that it cannot be taken for granted and that it is, in principle, endangered, he already addresses himself to a third person, whom precisely he wants to exclude. Why should someone who addresses himself exclusively to someone else specifically justify his address by stressing its exclusivity? The third, excluded person is no longer such a person. Could someone who addresses himself exclusively to someone else stress exclusivity at all? But if exclusive and excluding address turns out to be impossible from its inception, could one then say that the fiction of a general public is always inscribed in the address? The exclusive and excluding address of the activist is the self-contradictory attempt at unifying absolute difference and absolute control of meaning in the fiction of a particular public, which supposedly can be delimited in its particularity. This attempt is self-contradictory because the absolute control of the meaning of absolute difference crosses out both the differing and the meaning.[17]

The phenomenon of *outing* is directly linked to the questions of address and identity posed by activism in the time of AIDS; it is linked to questions that are also posed *to* activism, and that it attempts to answer. A justification for outing, which has the advantage of being unmistakable, is provided by activist Larry Kramer, initiator of ACT UP and founder of the organization GMHC (Gay Men's Health Crisis). Although one must keep in mind that Kramer's statement does not belong explicitly to the context of a discussion of outing, this hardly affects its suitability as a justification. Kramer claims apodictically: "It is now a truism that every gay man who stays in the closet is helping to kill the rest of his fellow gay men" (Kramer, p. 246). Outing as an aggressive affirmation of homosexuality, as a vindication of homosexual identity that directs itself against so-called "homophobia," turns into a retrospective action by means of which justice is to be done, after the fact, to what is irretrievably past. Revealing the secret avenges the murder. Not even those who died before the epidemic spread of AIDS are safe from a retrospective praxis of outing. The one who does the outing, and gets worked up all the more in the time of AIDS, behaves as if it were a matter of establishing solidarity with the suffering of past generations by, above all, enlightening them—particularly their prominent representatives—about their own suffering, which they have misunderstood. The flash of hope is not received from the past, but rather passed on to the past.

Rhetorically and ideologically trained, the North American literary critic D. A. Miller knows how to address contemporary and past generations. In an extensive review he analyzes and denounces the address structure noticeable in Susan Sontag's essay on AIDS. The "arrogant silence" of an author who wants to maintain distance is dictated, according to Miller, by the "general consciousness" of the public to which her analysis is addressed. But the involuntary effects of an "unconscious" that determines the "general consciousness" of Sontag's audience, as well as the form of address belonging to such a consciousness, allegedly betray the intellectual distance and the neutral objectivity as ideological trappings. Again, the question of address reveals itself as a question concerning the concepts of universality and the public (sphere). Miller concedes, however, that Sontag recognizes the veiling function that corresponds to the notion of a "general population" in the context of thinking and talking about AIDS (Miller [1], pp. 96–97). Sontag recognizes that this notion is, in truth, "a code phrase for whites as it is for heterosexuals" (p. 94). But her own thinking and talking about AIDS, Miller charges, are also addressed to a "pseudo-universal and -unified entity" (p. 96), to precisely that entity which Sontag occasionally calls the "general consciousness." Because the "unconscious" that accompanies consciousness contradicts the semblance of neutrality that this consciousness wants to produce, one must consider as decisive, for understanding the "general consciousness," that which this consciousness does not itself think, that is, its own "identification with the priorities of a transatlantic intelligentsia" (p. 99), to which Miller ascribes the attributes of a white skin and heterosexual orientation. Miller treats Sontag's text as a syndrome that must be identified in its complexity, but this method does not lead to the unfolding or further development of a thought. Identification and naming of the ever-same motifs, by which this complexity is represented as something fundamentally simple, turns out in the end to be merely an affirmation and confirmation of what one suspects anyway. The danger of such a critique, which castigates the "general consciousness" as a consciousness of "homophobia, racism, and cultural conservatism" (p. 100), consists in merely prolonging domination through its claim of unmasking dominating knowledge. Where enlightenment is reduced to the zealous practice of identifying, it becomes a ritual and mechanical action, prohibitive to independent thinking. Pure outing, however, is nothing other than such a prohibition of thinking.

How does one address and respond to things past? Miller's essay *Bringing out Roland Barthes*, intended to bring the semiologist out of the darkroom, is dedicated to a dead person. It is addressed to a dead person whose homosexuality must be brought out into the light of day because the person in question, as well as his "homophobic critics," still cover it up all too handily. Naturally, the outing happens with the best moral, political, and literary-theoretical

intentions. Only the performative act of "bringing out" makes le-
gitimate acts of stating possible, since the reception of Barthes's
works allegedly depends on it: "To refuse to bring Barthes out
consents to a homophobic reception of his work" (Miller [2], p.
7). Detective Miller, whose gaze is reproduced on the book cover
and presumably is meant to penetrate the eyes of the reader, uses
his method of unmasking in order to expose the secret that is no
secret. He accuses Barthes of a "quasi-paranoid mistrust" (p. 23), a
mistrust of all qualities and peculiarities that allegedly appear in
their "discernible gay specificity" (p. 16). The detective himself,
however, seems to have contracted just such a case of paranoia. Although Barthes rarely thematizes homosexuality explicitly, it im-
prints every treated topic with its decipherable and recognizable
signature, or so goes Miller's assumption, no matter how loose the
connection between the topic and homosexuality. The logic of an
unconscious compulsion to confess, on which Miller bases his argument, is disarmingly simple. It consists of three steps: the semiologist Barthes was homosexual; he let himself be intimidated by
scientific and academic institutions; therefore he condemned himself to talking incessantly about his homosexuality. Against his own
will, Barthes speaks in a "gay voice" (p. 25).[18]

Miller does recognize that the public display of a concealed "homosexual meaning," invisible at first sight, and the will to identification and control of meaning recall the methods of the police
used in hunting criminals. But this similarity in no way discour-
ages him in his intention: to write a long essay in which his own
contribution over wide stretches is limited to the application of
these methods. *Bringing out Roland Barthes* hardly contains an
original thought; it is instead characterized by a resentment that, to
quote Nietzsche, "from the beginning says 'No' to an 'outside,' to
an 'other,' to a 'not-self.'" Miller sees signs of a "homophobic con-
spiracy" everywhere; everything indicates only a homosexual meaning. While collecting, with detective-like zeal, alleged evidence that
he finds always and everywhere, Miller simultaneously acts as the
deadly serious and inexorable judge who heads the inquisition into

"men's gayness" in order to burn every *gaya scienza* at the stake. It is not without good reason that he neglects to reflect on the ambiguity to which he exposes himself when accusing Susan Sontag of an "intellectualization" of the epidemic (Miller [1], p. 99).[19]

In Miller one can read the repressive, authoritarian traits of *outing* or *bringing out*. Outing inevitably reproduces the structure of the revealed secret, and the piles supporting the foundation of the society of control in which we live are driven even deeper. Forcible revelation can, in certain cases, be a means of denouncing hypocrisy when hypocrisy serves an interest in holding on to power. It can thereby be an instrument for the subversion of power; it can be used against the interests that control society. But it becomes an instrument for the oppressive control of meaning when it is generalized and ideologically legitimated. In a courageous and insightful paper, Silvia Bovenschen pointed this out unequivocally: "Someone who refuses to render himself universally accessible and classifiable, even though according to general opinion he belongs to a type that may become the object of a discussion, is suspect. In outing he is categorically categorized. . . . This notorious skepticism about the lies that mark other lives thus aims at dogmatizing what one has found to be homosexual, true, and good about oneself. And, O wonder of revelation: the unmasked truth is what one has always already assumed it to be. . . . Even in what is other, otherness is not supposed to show its colors. Where would we end up if those similarly discriminated against did not, in the end, really resemble each other?" (Bovenschen, pp. 4–5) Outing is one more strategy of control.

Certainly, the activist's way of thinking identity does not take up strategies of control simply arbitrarily, but in the name of infected homosexuals, who are condemned to death by the arbitrary rule of the interests of state, economy, and science. And certainly it cannot be repeated often enough that it has been activism fighting against such interests that has so far effected the most important—indeed, the only—changes to which many infected and ill people owe their survival to this day. But the control of meaning that the activist's thinking of identity exerts, and must exert in order to prove itself as such, reproduces the repressive politics against which it stands up and which it justifiably denounces. The activist says, because I must not turn to a general—in truth, particular and exclusive—public, I address myself exclusively to a particular, limited, and identifiable public, which does not conceal its particularity, but flaunts it. It is as if the control of meaning (which here, for example, secures the possibility of its practice with a simple reversal of address) negated, denied, or repressed the danger of contagion: linguistic purity and purification, conjuration meant to stave off AIDS. Thus, a paradoxical consequence must be drawn from the activist's program: the exclusive and excluding address directed to the so-called "risk groups" immediately excludes these groups. In the final analysis, the activist thinks in the categories of exclusions, among which, after all, the category of "risk group" also belongs.

Perhaps at least a part of the activists' success derives from the fact that the strategies of activism *perpetuate* a reactionary politics of identity. Not-at-one with AIDS must therefore mean not-at-one with a politics of identity. However, not-at-one with AIDS also means this: Be-not-at-one with AIDS. Don't let yourself be intimidated by the politics of identity. Undertake everything to search for and invent modes of political intervention that cannot be justified by means of identity politics.[20] Who will protect the maxim "I am out; therefore I am"—meant to signify the constitution of an identity through a consciousness-raising, externalized expression, or a liberating, internalized recollection—from Being-not-one, from the *out* of a Being-not-one that is no longer opposed to an inside, and whose outside does not constitute a new inside? Who will guard addressing-oneself-to, which activism wants to control and transform into an act of controlling meaning, from im-pertinence?

If one addresses oneself to the general public, one addresses oneself to all and to everyone. If one addresses a particular public, one addresses this person and that person. To whom should one address oneself when talking about AIDS if the two spheres of a general and a particular public turn out to be politically dangerous fic-

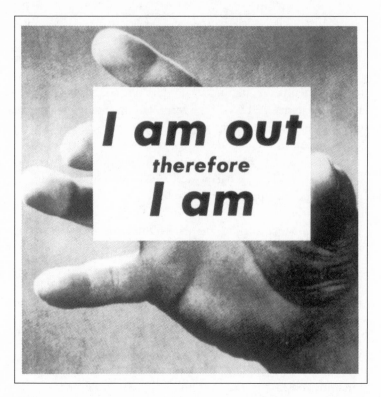

Fig. 2 Adam Rolston, *I Am Out; Therefore I Am*

tions of meaning control and of the thinking of identity, fictions of
exclusion and discrimination, of the reduction of Being-not-one
to a Being-one? Perhaps to everyone and no one.

Late in the evening across the park from west to east in a cab we
did not know anything about the accident on the empty street not yet
after the blow you dug your head into my arms that day I told you for
the first time about the mission with which I boarded the plane to find
a means for a painless quick suicide whom could I have asked if not
you from whom of course I could not ask advice the specialist in death
or discretion that makes you all the more silent I wished the impossible
for us TO JUST SAY EVERYTHING AND TO SAY IT SIMPLY *beyond the*

moods and without repercussions and reactions in unshakable nearly feelingless trust that resists all provocations call it love or friendship don't name it we would have thought and talked about the virus in the same way "ne jamais invoquer, ne pas laisser venir au langage les Noms, source de disputes, d'arrogances et de morales," never invoke or rely on something, never let the Names come to language, never let them speak, they are the source of dispute, of arrogance, and of morality.

Once the question of the *who*, of the address, of the addressees of thinking and talking about AIDS has been posed, one cannot help asking what happens in such an address, in such an addressing-oneself-to.

What happens in the process of thinking about AIDS? What distinguishes this thinking-about from just any reflection on just any object?

Judging from the pamphlets and articles of the activist Larry Kramer, one can understand thinking and talking about AIDS as testimony. The activist understands himself as a witness, that is, as someone who bears responsibility and fulfills a duty. Thinking and speaking become testimony only when the thinking and speaking subject is a responsible one who by thinking and speaking carries out a duty. That thinking and that talking become testimony that face the law—human, practical, divine, or mythical. "I felt I had an obligation," says Larry Kramer. "Because fate had placed me on the front line of this epidemic from the very beginning, I was a witness to much history that other writers were not" (Kramer, p. 145). Kramer invokes a dramatic and combative confrontation: an ideology of the writer as journalist is inscribed in his statements. The conjuring of historical simultaneity attaches in a mythical dependency to a principle of fate, which establishes coherence by delegating and privileging certain roles. Its function is to guarantee the credibility of the witness, the definite character of the testimony, and the identifiability of the report, of what is reported and of the one who reports. Such a historical simultaneity cannot be reduced to a historical condition; it is impossible to reduce the duty to which the reporting activist refers to nothing but a simple historical condition or fact. No testimony can originate in historical occurrences that exhaust themselves in themselves or in something that is not what they are, that is other. But if historical occurrences exist only to the extent that history exhausts itself neither in itself nor in another, testimony is not something added to history from the outside. Rather, testimony has its origin in the constitutive Being-not-one of history. If history exhausted itself in a pure sequence of contingent occurrences, then it would be indifference, which does not know testimony; it would be an accumulation of occurrences that could not even be perceived as such. If on the other hand history were absorbed in something super- or unhistorical, then it would be, as history, at most an occasion for having access to something different from historical events, not actually a historical occurrence about which testimony could be given. Thus, testimony and history are inextricably intertwined. Testimony is not simply another dimension of dealing with history. In other words, as little as a pure historiography free from all testimony can be thought—that is, a historiography that does not already cancel its object and thus weaken the ground on which it stands—just as little can one think a historical reflection in the course of which history becomes the occasion for an unhistorical meditation, for meditation on something that is elevated above or excepted from history. Such a reflection, absolute testimony, erases the occasion that it requires. It does not give testimony; it gives itself up.

The non-historical is not a concept that is juxtaposed to the historical, a definite unity that sublates the historical or a substance foreign to history. It is, if at this point one may still use these terms, history as Being-not-one, as Being-not-one without determination and without sublation. History is more than or other than an occasion, a negativity, an indifferent collection of facts, because, not-one with itself, never itself, and therefore non-historical, it incessantly exposes and interrupts any positing. It opens up anything that has come about, that has fossilized, that has closed itself off, splitting the opening itself: history is neither a closed totality nor a pure opening to a substantialized other. Instead of entering a speculative vision of history by letting itself be identified as a historical rupture, the emergence of AIDS, which so far knows no limits, makes visible this originary Being-not-one of history, a Being-not-one that can never appear as a phenomenon. Perhaps testimony is not what it is supposed to be: that which makes possible the retrospective definition of an incident or accident, of an unusual event-like occurrence[21] through attesting that something definite and specific has happened, or is about to happen. Rather, testimony is the mark of originary Being-not-one. But why can such a marking be called testimony? How does such marking testimony come about? What exactly constitutes the testimony of Being-not-one? Of what does the duty, the responsibility, of the witness consist who thinks and talks about AIDS?

That the understanding of the historical can never be reduced to a registering, constructing, determining, and defining knowledge, in short: to scientific knowledge; that historical understanding is essentially dependent on something that cannot be overtaken by, and remains incompatible with, knowledge; that, on the other hand, it should not be regarded as something contingent or vanishing, a mere occasion for the discovery of "the truth that I had from the beginning without knowing it" (Kierkegaard, p. 12): this is the thought Kierkegaard attempts to unfold in his *Philosophical Fragments.* The historical is a contradiction, and therefore already not-one with itself. It is always the past; as the past, it has a reality; that it happened proves certain, according to Kierkegaard. Historiography that aims at comprehension is perhaps motivated precisely by such a certainty, even if it has to overlook the contradiction that separates certainty from itself and exposes it to uncertainty. For precisely in the certainty of the having-occurred one must notice the uncertainty that constantly hinders us from comprehending the historical, that which has come about; this uncertainty prevents us from identifying the historical as something that has been "from eternity" (Kierkegaard, p. 79). Thus Kierkegaard points out that every comprehension, all scientific knowledge, of history already misses history, because defining and identifying necessarily transform the identified and defined into necessity. Historical becoming is dehistoricized and neutralized by identification and definition. The historical decays into a mere occasion for something super- or ahistorical; it becomes the occasion for necessity to manifest itself. "Only in this contradiction between certainty and uncertainty, the *discrimen* [distinctive mark] of something that has come into existence and thus also of the past, is the past understood" (ibid.). Only the contradiction of the historical, that is, its certain uncertainty and its uncertain certainty, renders the occurrences historical, thus distinguishing them from the ahistorical indifference of pure contingency and pure necessity. But even the distinguishing itself, the discrimination of which Kierkegaard speaks, must be touched by the Being-not-one of the contradiction if it is not to reintroduce necessity through the back door. In the instant that Being-not-one assumes the identifiable form of a contradiction, the stability of a discriminating, distinguishing criterion is reestablished. That which is distinguished is identified anew; history is again submitted to a unity, and uncertainty appears, at best, as a lack of certainty, as a provisional uncertainty. The Being-not-one of history asserts itself in the impossibility of determining a stable and certain criterion, a *discrimen* that permits making a distinction between history and the nonhistorical.

If the knowledge that is associated with a comprehending historiography or with a philosophy of history dehistoricizes historical occurrences, one must find ways to relate to history other than through comprehension or determination. Something incommensurable with identification, with thinking that defines and comprehends, is inscribed in definition and comprehension, which originate in the certainty of what has happened while trying to create this very certainty. An incommensurable element is inscribed in the defining and comprehending thought of identification, because the certainty of what has to be comprehended and defined is itself split by an indefinite and incomprehensible uncertainty. This incommensurable other Kierkegaard calls "belief" or "faith": "It is clear, then, that the organ for the historical must be formed in

likeness to this, must have within itself the corresponding something by which in its certitude it continually sublates the incertitude that corresponds to the uncertainty of coming into existence.
Such uncertainty is a double uncertainty: it is the uncertainty of
the nothingness of non-being and the uncertainty of annihilated
possibility, which is also the annihilation of every other possibility. This is precisely the nature of belief or faith, for continually
present as the sublated in the certitude of belief is the incertitude
that in every way corresponds to the uncertainty of coming into
existence" (Kierkegaard, p. 81). The dialectical discourse on sublation and on the presence of what is sublated should not lead us
merely to find comfort in the sublation of uncertainty and overlook possibilities for radicalizing Kierkegaard's argument.[22] For if
belief were nothing but a certainty that sublated uncertainty, as
thinking sublates negativity, one could indeed distinguish between
the certainty of belief and the truth of thinking, but ultimately belief and faith would only set the scene for or complement thinking.

In Kierkegaard, belief is not added to the historical from the
outside. Nor does belief complement a historical comprehension
that must lack the unity of the concept. Rather, belief is historical
behavior itself, the only behavior that does justice to history, that
is, if one can ever do justice to history and if there is a historical
behavior that can be distinguished as such. Not the least consequence of Kierkegaard's argument is that one can bring it to bear
independently of its Christian-theological articulation. Everything
Kierkegaard says about belief and witnessing can be generalized,
because to the degree that it follows from the meditation on the
Being-not-one of history it is not in need of dogmatic presupposi-
tions and conversion. The meditation on the Being-not-one of history demonstrates that one can relate to history only if one has experience of belief, only if experience is determined, as it were, by
an experience of belief. This, however, is not to say that one has to
believe in something determinate or definite, in a definite content
of belief. The definite content of belief—the interpretation of Being-not-one in the spirit of a paradoxical "eternalizing of the historical" and "historicizing of the eternal" (p. 61)—is exposed to

uncertainty by Kierkegaard's own description: "The faith that celebrates triumphantly is the most ludicrous thing of all" (p. 108). As the paradox of thinking, as the general passion of thought, faith affords no security against the undoing of understanding, no hold to which the individual can cling. The person whose understanding is in danger of foundering must endure the uncertainty of belief and faith. In this sense, faith is not just the stabilizing supplement of thinking. Kierkegaard's analysis exposes the *discrimen* to the non-discriminable; because of its irreducible im-pertinence, it can be nothing other than a discontinuous, discrete collection of philosophical pieces, which never vouch for their universality. At the same time, there is no doubt that Kierkegaard claims a certain universality for his analysis, even if this claim is itself uncertain: "This, then, is the ultimate paradox of thought: to want to discover something that thought itself cannot think. This passion of thought is fundamentally present everywhere in thought, also in the single individual's thought insofar as he, thinking, is not merely himself" (p. 37). If one were now to consider faith as a consequence of thinking that has become entangled in an unsolvable paradox, if one were now to consider faith to be a paradox of thinking from which one can draw consequences, then one would entirely misunderstand faith and dissolve the paradox: "But, humanly speaking, consequences built upon a paradox are built upon the abyss, and the total content of the consequences, which is handed down to the single individual only under the agreement that it is by virtue of a paradox, is not passed down like a sheltered inheritance, since the whole thing is in suspension" (p. 98). The paradox must be experienced anew every time. It can never be accepted or passed on as a secured condition of faith or belief. Thus, the specific content of faith or belief and the interpretation of Being-not-one as "historicizing of the eternal" and "eternalizing of the historical" can never display the firm shape of inherited dogma, of a possession or a good that can be handed down.

One cannot rely on the paradox in order to justify faith or belief. Therefore, faith or belief is tied to the moment of decision. It is not a decisionism, not an arbitrary act of deciding, that is manifest in Kierkegaard's recourse to the concept of decision, but the Being-not-onė of history, which of course does not make itself known as a manifestation: "This casts light on belief also. When belief resolves to believe, it runs the risk that it was an error, but nevertheless it wills to believe. One never believes in any other way; if one wants to avoid risk, then one wants to know with certainty that one can swim before going into the water" (p. 83). The act of deciding, with which one steps not "out" of history but rather "into" it, "into" Being-not-one—otherwise the moment is again transformed into a mere pretext—is different from the decisionist act of a subject, since the consistency of an act of will presupposes the constitution of a thinking or believing subjectivity. The non-decisionist, non-subjective act of decision, which is historical in its divided certainty and which Kierkegaard calls the act of faith ("although for us it is not a matter of the name"), is—in its radicalization—the act of testifying. It is the act of testifying that is in each case unique and in each case a repetition, a performative without knowledge, that does not testify to anything definite and that resists definition.

Thus, one becomes a witness only when one can no longer rely on knowledge and when testimony, which evades identification, does not testify to any definite something but must nevertheless relate to a series of occurrences that is in itself not-one. Because testimony does not hand down any knowledge (not even knowledge about the faith of the witness), the contemporaneity of a witness with an occurrence, the immediacy of witnessing, the historical eyewitness's reliability—emphasizing this reliability is meant to point to "absolutely exact historical knowledge" (p. 59)—can only divert the attention of a non-contemporary, the member of a later generation; it cannot serve as the basis for charges about "whether he [the contemporary] actually had the faith that he testified he had" (p. 102). Does not the concept of witness as such contain an irreducible non-contemporaneity and non-simultaneity, without which it would not seem meaningful at all to speak of and be in need of a witness? Absolute simultaneity excludes witnessing.

Of course, at this point ("to have *the* faith") one could object that Kierkegaard still subscribes too much to dialectics in order to clear the way for a radicalization of his thought. Insofar as he interprets Being-not-one as the dialectic of the historical and the eternal, insofar as the moment thus collects, accumulates, concentrates, capitalizes, in itself the "fullness of time" (p. 18); insofar as time is meant to touch the eternal in the moment;[23] insofar as the condition of faith, which is "provided" (p. 59) by the paradox, conditions an interpretation of Being-not-one, faith that gives testimony is endowed with content and stability. Thus, one will always be able to say that Kierkegaard's exposing [*Aussetzung*] of faith and belief is always their investiture [*Einsetzung*], and that uncertainty is subjected to certainty. The more Kierkegaard exposes faith or understands exposure as faith, the more strongly he exposes history to its constitutive Being-not-one, the more fervor he invests in the investiture of faith and the more he dehistoricizes historical occurrences. Perhaps relevant in this context is a formulation that presents the paradox as *that which unites* the contradictory elements. The contradiction is thus submitted to a unity; the non-simultaneous, dissimilar, uneven simultaneity of mutually exclusive occurrences is transposed into a unifying present, and the paradox is dissolved. "But the paradox specifically *unites* the contradictories," writes Kierkegaard. "[It] is the eternalizing of the historical and the historicizing of the eternal" (p. 61; my emphasis).

To destabilize the stabilized act of faith—the testimony of Christian dogma to God's having become human—it perhaps suffices to point out that this unification, this stabilization, this dehistorization, is a matter of an interpretation that does not necessarily follow from a reading of the *Philosophical Fragments* that takes seriously the idea of uncertainty. To object that one could also claim that the meditations of the *Philosophical Fragments* acquire their meaning only through the fact that they stand in a horizon created by dogma does not hold, because then the entire approach of these meditations would turn out to be questionable: the distinction between the Socratic and the Christian, the occasion and the moment, knowledge and belief, would be invalidated.

Faith, interpreted as "belief in," is already an interpretation of faith—of faith that never discloses itself to knowledge, that is not something knowable, or a virtual knowledge. Testimony as the mark of originary Being-not-one, which can be identified neither *as* the historical nor *as* the non-historical, also testifies to the danger of turning non-knowledge into knowledge, faith into a "belief in." But one thus faces two questions: if the dogma is shattered in its inception, if it seems that a defined faith or a determinate belief is reduced to a simple believing, to an acceptance without a final proof of what has been accepted, what, then, entitles us to speak of a testimony and an experience of faith, of a duty to testify and a responsibility to give testimony? How can testimony come about, a behavior or an action that marks Being-not-one and thus distinguishes it from the indifference of purely contingent, arbitrary, indistinguishable occurrences?

Giving testimony comes about because Being-not-one does not engender an immanence closed in itself, but rather—with every interruption, every discontinuity, every crisis—creates space for a behavior, for an adhering-to-oneself, which conducts itself in relation to that which does not engender orderly relations. Giving testimony comes about because mere believing, as acceptance, is meant to correspond to the essential instability of Being-not-one, but is ultimately only a form of knowledge, even if it is a weak form. A non-dogmatic experience of faith should not be confused with believing as acceptance. Giving testimony comes about because no immediate contemporaneity with historical occurrences can be produced, that is, no immediate simultaneity with Being-not-one. Kierkegaard emphasizes that the immediate contemporary is most likely to succumb to the semblance of a privileged access to occurrences and thus to deprive himself of the experience of faith as an experience of history. Giving testimony comes about because Being-not-one must be marked and thus time and again distinguished from knowledge and "belief in," which usurp it: the possibility of such a usurpation is the origin of the duty and responsibility to testify, in a way that is not responsible for something determined and not obligated to a determinable instance.

Giving testimony comes about because there can no more be a communication of what is testified to than there can be any simultaneity with Being-not-one. Giving testimony does not communicate anything: it has no communicable content. It does not testify to anything definite that could be handed down in the form of a content; it does not tell a story or history; no historiography can rely on it. Perhaps in the time of AIDS a way of giving testimony, a marking of Being-not-one, comes about that communicates nothing and erases itself because such a paradoxical marking must always also be understood as the attempt to exhibit Being-not-one *as such*. Only when this exhibition is thought can one perhaps speak of a duty and a responsibility to give testimony.

Is it possible to imagine a thinking and talking about AIDS, an activism, that gives testimony of Being-not-one with AIDS? *Reactive* activism gives testimony of the epidemic by subscribing to the telling of its fateful story and by acting in the service of a (collective) subject. This activism conceals, denies, or negates Being-not-one only to be content, in the name of a rhetorical-practical politics of identity, with a negative Being-not-at-one. *Active* activism, on the other hand, sees its task as marking and giving testimony of Being-not-one, as a preparation for a life that depends only on the possibility of exhibiting Being-not-one as such and consists precisely of this exhibition, of this always uncertain, never secured transformation of the fragmentary, equivocal, obscure, aporetic, unsolvable, and indistinguishable.

With my heart pounding I stood in the elevator of the old highrise on Lexington Avenue and thought it was a miracle that I even came this far, nobody stopped me, although they would have had to carry me outside at first glance, your forgetting is the protection from forgetting with which my memory punishes you, it would not be forgetting if I did not time and again want to transform it, in despair, because it challenges me incessantly, I have to work to exhaustion on the memory that I would like to keep open for your forgetting, that is meant to attract it and to be loved by it unconditionally, no, you don't want any effort and you despise any effort with which I want to touch you finally I am supposed to follow your forgetting to love it without ever requesting from you that you turn around tired and reconciled because of the exhaustion, what I call your silence is my last bastion, you despise my desire to still find my way in it, you live in another world to which I have no entry.

One may try to address everyone and no one while thinking and talking about AIDS. One may test forms of an active activism, which in thinking, talking, and action give testimony, a testimony with neither a determined nor a determinable content. Another question, however, imposes itself upon us:

How is one to think and talk about AIDS, how is one to act without being overwhelmed and paralyzed by the extent of the epidemic, the number of the dead, the disease or death of a beloved person in whose blood the virus circulates?

On the one hand, activism stresses that one must not lose any time in mourning, that too much time is lost that way. One does not have the time necessary for the work of mourning, because one would have to mourn too much and because the mourning seems to destroy its own economy of time: mourning becomes infinite and thus impossible. It succumbs to its own overexertion, its exhaustion, its extension beyond itself, beyond all boundaries (Kramer, p. 222). The question is not whether a complete work of mourning can ever be performed but whether mourning is possible at all, for the shortest period of mourning already diverts one from the urgent tasks of practice. Activism is in danger of turning into its opposite, quietism, when it grants time to mourning and its public manifestations—the so-called "candlelight marches," the numerous mourning and memorial observances (pp. 264–65).[24] From such a point of view, therefore, the work of mourning always lasts too long. Mourning's economy of time poses a danger to activism, a distraction that affects its very possibility. Thus it is only consistent that the reflection which might be triggered by the experience of mourning is equally dismissed by activists: "Death as a profound philosophical subject is currently ridiculous" (p. 222). Because one cannot afford to mourn, one is also unable to think about death. The impossibility of mourning extends itself to contemplation and reflection, to thinking about death. Thinking about death is thus made impossible, and so is the thinking and mourning about the impossibility of this thinking. The proper names in newspaper obituaries are integrated into that mechanical memory which in speculative philosophy is already supposed to suit proper names. How, then, does the practice of activism differ from a mechanism? Is not the twofold impossibility of mourning and reflection—which activism establishes and propagates so that it will not be forced to abandon the possibility and the identity of activist action[25]—precisely the impossibility of such action, that is, the impossibility of a practice of intervention and change?

On the other hand, activism laments the lack of a philosophy of death and of finitude, even the overall lack of a philosophical thinking to help people with AIDS. For the activist Gregg Bordowitz, nothing is more important than talking about the lack of *a* philosophy or the lack *of* philosophy (Caruth and Keenan, p. 552). It is as if activism split into the two (identical) extremes of anti-intellectualism and hyper-intellectualization but simultaneously pointed out an aporia that cannot be detached from Being-not-one with AIDS. Crimp recognizes that activist resistance to mourning depends on how one assesses and interprets AIDS. That is, it depends on whether one sees the "crisis" as either a "natural, accidental catastrophe," which happens at a definite point in time, or as the result of "gross political negligence," an occurrence, that is, which has been made possible, tolerated, and until now endured (Crimp, p. 6).[26] In order to resist the simplification contained in such interpretations, in order to make clear the reduction that lies in the assessment of mourning to which these interpretations might lead, Crimp tries to produce a different connection between "mourning and militancy." From the perspective of his investigation, mourning and militant practice do not exclude each other. On the contrary, mourning transforms itself into militant practice. Both "profound mourning" and "melancholia," to use Freud's terms, call forth a "turning away from any activity not connected with the memory of the deceased" (Freud [3], p. 244/198). The "normal" work of mourning, however, amounts to a "reality-test-ing," which makes sure that "respect for reality gains the day." In the end, the ego ought to behave in a "free and uninhibited" way. It is precisely this testing of reality—Freud counts it among the "major institutions of the ego"—which, according to Crimp, turns the one who mourns into an activist. But "respect for reality" does not simply triumph, for it is inseparable from a struggle against the established order and its reality. Consequently, activism feeds on, perpetuates, the work of mourning to the degree that it pre-vents the victory of reality, of the established order. Thus, mourn-ing does not juxtapose itself against activism; it does not paralyze militancy. Rather, activism that does not repress death is essen-tially a work of mourning. To put it differently: the individual work of mourning leads, in the shape of activism, to the collective work of mourning. A successful, "normal" activist work of mourn-ing would have changed reality, would have engendered a reality that withstands the critical test: "*I am out; therefore I am.*"

Crimp, whose translation of a metapsychological analysis of the "normal affect of mourning" into concepts of collectivity and uni-versality also relies on Freud,[27] is aware of the difficulties for a pol-itics of identity that are associated with the activist's work of mourning. Each instance of mourning is not just mourning for a dead person but for the "ideal" of "gay sexuality," for homosexu-ality as such (Crimp, p. 11). This is the case, at least, if the identity of homosexuals and of homosexuality is defined by such an ideal, an ideal whose power of abstraction is not unrelated to the mo-ment of abstraction that adheres to promiscuity and to the epi-demic that ends such promiscuity.[28] For activism to be a work of mourning, for mourning and militancy not to exclude each other, an ideal, an idealizing power of abstraction, must be involved. The (activist's) work of mourning requires "identification" (Crimp, p. 9) with the dead in order "to withdraw all libido from its attach-ments to the object" (Freud [3], p. 244/198). But this identifica-tion turns out to be problematic for the success of the work of mourning and of the activist's actions, for it exposes the possibility of living *on*—the replacement of the libido position that has been given up—to the narcissism of *out*living. Dangerous contagion: "living on" means surviving, means turning a narcissistic profit from living on—a profit that actually cannot be turned and that is inseparable from feelings of guilt. Because in each case one mourns the ideal, one leads the existence of a specter. Insofar as one oriented oneself to the ideal, one can accuse oneself of murder[29]—of the killing of the other and the destruction of the ideal, the ideal without which there is no other and without which one irretrievably loses one's own identity. With the dissolution of identity, however, readiness to reproach oneself also vanishes. It is no longer even possible to speak of reproaching oneself and to say that this reproaching is evidence of a transition from mourning to melancholy. The melancholy condition presupposes a love-object that can be recognized and a loving, mourning subject: "The loss of a love-object," Freud says, "is an excellent opportunity for the ambivalence in love-relationships to make itself effective and come into the open. Where there is a disposition to obsessional neurosis the conflict due to ambivalence gives a pathological cast to mourning and forces it to express itself in the form of self-reproaches to the effect that the mourner himself is to blame for the loss of the loved object, i.e., that he has willed it" (Freud [3], pp. 250–51/204). In the time of AIDS, which seems to demand a politics of identity and of the ideal, gay activism as a work of mourning is an enterprise that due to its internal contradictions can hardly be sustained.

The loss of the ideal, the destruction of identity, and the paralyzing of the "institutions of the ego" interrupt any possible work of mourning. But perhaps we should not—as activists believe who are still too influenced by a politics of identity—provide new philosophical projects or dress up old systems of thought with (post-)modernist facades. As soon as philosophy is assigned such a task, it is reduced to being a reactive *Weltanschauung* and not much more can be expected from it than the ideological putty used to repair old structures. Philosophy must itself have an active function. Does not the philosophical-political act consist in an intervention, a change of perspective that can never be entirely overtaken by arguments and that is made possible by the interruption of the work of mourning and the (activist) politics of identity? This change, which does not simply replace one perspective by a different perspective, happens when one becomes aware of the possibility of an originary Being-not-one, or of an im-pertinent existence. An im-pertinent existence does not carry out any work of mourning, not because it is indifferent to disease and death, not because it declares death and disease to be mere appearance, or because it seeks deliverance in them, but because its relation to both is of another kind. The question of an im-pertinent existence is the question of a relation to sickness and death that distinguishes itself essentially from the work of mourning, from the perpetuation of the complex of melancholia, and from the idealizing denial of what has been endured.[30]

I wanted to know what these objects were called and I received the answer Día de los muertos-things *a little box open at the front like a small stage and the strangest of all scenes not simply a moralizing one with skull and legend like the others but two small figures made out of clay naked men with erect penises turning their backs to each other in the shower their gaze seems to be fixed on the tiled wall a mirror behind them reflects their bodies.*

§ 4 Recognizing the Virus

Thesis for a prospective assessment: It will have been said about AIDS that it makes visible that which always already determines our thinking and action—without our knowing it.

On January 22, 1990, Julien Green notes a brief story in his diary: "I was told about a young man who is HIV-positive and has known about his infection for about two years; Catholic friends take it upon themselves to convert him since he is completely unbelieving. The case is not simple: as hard as he tries, the patient cannot find his way to belief. He just smiles and says no. His friends, even more obstinate, do not give up. Several months pass. Time and again they pray for him. One day the young man says to his best friend, 'I've written a poem.' This is the gist of it: the young man goes for a walk and gets lost. A voice speaks to him: 'Give me your hand.' Answer: 'No.' He walks on without knowing where the path leads. Again the voice speaks to him: 'Give me your hand.' Again: 'No.' And he walks on. A third time, a hand reaches out to him, and the young man takes it. His friend asks him, 'What will the poem's title be?' The young man answers: 'God'" (Green, p. 547). What entitles us today to justify AIDS as a test that has the power to convert us to divine faith? Does such a justification not already contain the possibility of viewing AIDS as a punishment from God? Doesn't declaring AIDS a test or a trial, or acknowledging it as such, suffice to ascribe to the epidemic the meaning of a punishment or an opportunity, that is, the meaning of a possible restitution of meaning? Does such a production of meaning not suffice to derive a certain benefit from the epidemic?[1] Perhaps the question of what might warrant such an apology cannot be answered in a way that can be discursively articulated, at least not if we draw the consequences of what Jean-Luc Nancy says about the "death of God," namely, that neither use, nor profit, nor advantage of any kind can be gained from it. It is "unexploitable." "One takes note of it. One thinks *after* the death of God. That is all," Nancy states. The death of God is an event that must be taken note of, that must be acknowledged. Perhaps it even could be maintained that with the death of God death or finitude itself happens, if such a thing is possible. As soon as God dies, however, his death has become an immemorial event. The death of God remains unexploitable. We can only take note of it. We can only take note of the impossibility of deriving a benefit from it, of the impossibility of its exploitation, because this event cannot be brought to presence. The death of God is an event that does not have the characteristics of a historical moment. If it indicates anything at all, it is probably the impossibility of distinguishing event from structure, which is the paradoxical origin, the event-like "always-already" of history, structure, and discourse. The death of God happens; in the instant it happens, however, it has already happened and already determines that thinking which thinks after the event and merely takes note of it. Thus, this taking-note turns out to be an (impossible) experience *of* the impossible. One takes note of God's death, because one can think only after it; at the same time, however, there is nothing of which note can be taken, since in the instant of its happening, God's death has always already happened and has always already been noticed. To think after the death of God: one thinks about the death of God, about an event; one's own thoughts follow the dead or murdered God; one thinks because God's death has always already happened and God never died and was never murdered. But precisely this (impossible) experience of the impossible, of which this taking-note consists, also determines the relation to divine faith, as can be seen from the quoted diary entry.

The friend of the HIV-infected man can only take note of the title of the poem—and thus of the conversion. In other words, as one can think only after the death of God—because it can only be noticed, and it turns out to be, in the process of this noticing, what has always already been noticed—so one can only take note of divine faith and think only after the conversion. In this process too, the conversion itself becomes an immemorial event, which precedes thinking. Every attempt to provide a reason that might allow us to justify AIDS as a test of faith, every attempt to provide a reason that might prevent us from doing so, here encounters an insurmountable barrier.

In his essay "The Word of Nietzsche: 'God is Dead'" (1943), Heidegger seems to point to the problematic connection between thinking and a noticing that is always prior to it. On the one hand, the death of God is more than simply an opinion of a philosopher. Therefore, note must be taken of it. On the other hand, it is not an isolated, detachable event, but something that in a certain way has "always already" happened. If one takes note of it, it is simply because so far the pronouncement or the word "God is dead" has been said or made "without being spoken." But Heidegger does not simply think after the death of God. He comprehends the pronouncement "God is dead" as the truth of metaphysics, which is itself still unthought and can be thought only after the articulation of what was said without being spoken: "One could suppose that the pronouncement 'God is dead' expresses an opinion of Nietzsche the atheist and is accordingly only a personal attitude; one could suppose that it is one-sided, and easily refutable through the observation that today and in the whole world many men frequent the houses of God, enduring hardships out of a trust in God as defined by Christianity. But the question remains whether the aforesaid word of Nietzsche is merely an extravagant view of a thinker about whom the correct assertion is readily at hand: he finally went mad. And it remains to ask whether Nietzsche does not rather pronounce here the word that, within the metaphysically determined history of the West, has *always already* been said without being spoken" (Heidegger [4], p. 57/196; my emphasis). By equating the unspoken death of God with the unthought truth of metaphysics, Heidegger opens up a space in which this truth is yet to be thought and "God is dead" is yet to be spoken or repeated. It must be spoken or repeated as a metaphysically true pronouncement. Because there is a truth of truth, a truth of metaphysical truth, because the metaphysical truth is a happening, an event of truth that presupposes the event [*Ereignis*], but does not think its quality as an event, Heidegger's unfolding of a necessity, which elevates the pronouncement of God's death above mere opinion or conviction, implies a deferral of the question about that thinking which must take note of what it has always already taken note of— of what it has taken note of before it was even capable of taking note of it. Such a deferral can have a double function.

1. It can have a preparatory function. Heidegger concludes his treatise by declaring that the "madman," who proclaims the death of God in Nietzsche, searches and cries for God: "And the ear of our thinking? Does it still not hear the cry?" (p. 112/246). This preparatory function of the deferral can even be interpreted in such a way that the task of accomplishing the "foundation of the truth of Being," for which the last of the gods is waiting, is assigned to the thinking of the unthought truth of metaphysics—to the thinking that repeats the pronouncement "God is dead" because it has finally been uttered. In the *Contributions to Philosophy* Heidegger says, "The last god has his most singular singularity and stands outside of any calculating determination that is meant by the titles 'Mono-theism,' 'Pan-theism,' and 'A-theism.' 'Mono-theism' and all types of 'theism' have come about only since the Judeo-Christian 'apologetics,' which are the presupposition of 'metaphysics.' With the death of God all theisms fall into pieces" (Heidegger [5], p. 411). A few pages later, at the end of the chapter about the "last god," one reads the decisive passage: "How few know that the god is waiting for the foundation of the truth of Being. . . . Instead it seems that man would wait, and would have to

wait, for the god. Perhaps this is the most insidious form of the deepest godlessness" (p. 417). The god's waiting is a waiting for a transformation of beings "into the essentiality of their determination," which frees them of "machinations." Only when beings no longer exhaust themselves in a utilization or manipulation that makes them produce benefits, the moment for the "passing-by" of the last god arrives. Does this not mean that the waiting and the passing-by of the last god—of the god who comes after the death of God—remains alien to manipulation and that one therefore can gain no use and no benefit from the waiting and the passing-by? The circumstance that thinking prepares the passing-by of the last god, that the last god is waiting for this founding preparation, cannot be of use for thinking without its falling into "godlessness."

2. The deferral of the question, however, might also have the function of insisting on the heterogeneity of the relation between thinking and faith, of the radical difference between the two; thus it might have the function of securing the independence of each. The proceedings of the *Evangelische Akademie Hofgeismar* of 1953 give a synopsis of a conversation with Heidegger and contain a statement that clearly distinguishes the claim of faith from the determination of thinking. Within thinking, Heidegger maintains, nothing shall be accomplished that prepares or contributes to the determination of matters of faith. Distinguishing thinking from matters of faith, insisting on an essential alterity, is again an ambiguous gesture. It can either indicate that the question concerning God is deferred or that the death of God precedes thinking, that one thinks because one is able to think solely after the death of God. The event that one must understand this death to be cannot be made present through thought; one has to take note of it, one has to have an impossible experience of the impossible; the death of God, not conversion to divine belief, grants thinking its independence, so that it neither prepares the coming of the waiting god nor justifies faith. From this point of view, from the perspective of thinking, the distinction and the heterogeneity between the dimensions not only differentiate faith from thought, but amount to an obliteration of faith.

One may take note of the death of God or of conversion to divine faith; following the path of thinking, one may pave a way for the coming god or say nothing about such a coming. In each case, one has always already taken note of something that cannot be taken note of and that exceeds discursive justification. Only because it exceeds discursive justification was it possible to take note of it in an impossible experience of the impossible. Being-not-one and Being-not-at-one with AIDS also mean, as the discussion about the interpretation of the epidemic makes clear, that thinking and talking about the virus can never be completely recuperated and justified by discursive or purely argumentative means. When talking and thinking, one should be aware of this constitutive incompleteness and of this bound that opens the discourse to persuasion. One should be aware of it as much as possible.

But how does the emergence and spread of AIDS present itself to a thinking that takes note of the death of God and that thinks after it? How is AIDS thought by a thinking that thinks only to the extent to which the posteriority of this death—a peculiar posteriority that precedes itself—is constitutive for it? Nancy alludes to the emergence and spread of AIDS within the context of a sketchily outlined history of evil. He describes three ages, epochs, or periods of such a history and argues that today we find ourselves within evil itself. We no longer suffer evil in the form of an accident that befalls us (a tragic and definitive rupture, which is, however, still meaningful); neither do we experience it as sickness (as a rupture that permits reparation because "classical thought thinks before the backdrop of the disappearance or effacement of death"). The evil with which the history of evil reaches its end, the evil in the middle of which we are, evil itself, "does not come from the outside but originates with man." It resists reparation, it is definitive, and it cancels every possibility of meaning. Nancy situates AIDS within the context of this historical evil, which today no longer manifests itself as a (curable) illness: "In our eyes, AIDS does not come from God, but because it cannot yet be cured, it is seen as a sort of self-destruction of a society at the mercy of its own pure immanence" (Nancy [2], p. 29). From this perspective, the emergence and epidemic spread of AIDS raise the question of technology and its relation to freedom. If technology, on the one hand, designates an immanence without transcendence, or more precisely, if it designates that "there is neither immanence nor transcendence" (Nancy [3], p. 45), evil, on the other hand, must be understood as "a positive possibility of existence"; it is freedom, but a freedom "that unleashed turns against itself" (Nancy [4], p. 164). Here Nancy is in accord with Schelling's doctrine of freedom.

Clarifying the relationships among evil, freedom, and technology might provide us with conceptual means to think the emergence and spread of AIDS, because it allows us to take into account a *statement* and a *demand*. Thus, the historian Grmek *states* that "the AIDS epidemic came into being" due to "the technological upheaval of the modern world" (Grmek, p. xi/6). It is as if we had to confront a "perverse effect" of that which ought to bring about the end of diseases: "Contemporary technology could cause 'new' diseases, not only through degradation of the natural environment by all sorts of pollutants but also through methods designed to make living conditions more 'hygienic'" (p. 107/184). Bounan, for his part, *demands* that one obey particular "rules of hygiene," which are "incompatible with present social conditions." Such rules, therefore, "can only be obeyed completely if these conditions are overthrown (abolition of the commodity, of enslaving labor, of the State), and the general causes of the epidemic are thus removed: pollution, chemical fertilizers, social relations determined by the model of the commodity, the medicine of the marionette" (Bounan, p. 148). Bounan uses the expression "medicine of the marionette" to denounce a science that, according to its model of humanity, transforms human beings into "marionettes with souls"; it is a science opposed to a science that attempts to integrate men into a "living totality."

Once we have inscribed this statement and this demand into the conceptual framework that can be constructed following Nancy's arguments, and when we have reached a certain overview in this way, we still have to ask ourselves whether the history of evil, of which Nancy speaks in very general terms, exhausts itself in a progressive revelation of evil; that is, whether the emergence and epidemic spread of AIDS is but a form of this revelatory process that ends with the appearance of evil itself. How did the unleashing of freedom, which turning against itself inaugurates the history of evil, determine the development of a technology that in its essential diversity is always originary, delivering us perpetually into the non-immanent immanence of a finite existence? What exactly called forth the emergence of AIDS? What led to this revelation that seems always already programmed wherever evil is a positive possibility of existence? And if the death of God stands for a "first material extension of the world of bodies," if the word "God is dead" means that God "no longer has a body" (Nancy [5], pp. 53 and 55), how do the body and its extension relate to the evil of self-destruction, to self-destructing evil? How do they relate to the spread of AIDS, which is perceived as the evil of a technological immanence, of an immanence without transcendence and without immanence?

AIDS is always already inscribed in the program, is always already programmed and is always already on the program, that is, on the agenda. Another thinking resonates with these formulations, a thinking associated with the name Derrida. Along with Nancy, Jacques Derrida is probably one of the few philosophers or thinkers to inquire into the meaning of AIDS and remind us of the urgency of this question. He does so in an interview entitled "The Rhetoric of Drugs." In a different interview, responding to Nancy's question "Who comes after the subject?," Derrida expresses his wish to talk about AIDS and immediately adds that for him the emergence and spread of the virus represents an event [*Ereignis*]: "an event that one could call *historical* in the *epoch* of *subjectivity*, if we still gave credence to *historicality*, to *epochality*, and to *subjectivity*" (Derrida [3], p. 285/112). What does this curious statement tell us? On the one hand, we no longer give credence to the concepts Derrida enumerates; we no longer consider them creditworthy; we distrust them; we are not willing to support them and to be supported by them. On the other hand, we continue to credit them; their value still remains high enough; we believe that, despite their loss of credit, they might contribute to clarification of what AIDS challenges us to think. The emergence and spread of AIDS, then, is not an event. Or rather, it is an event because it is not a *pure* event. If we can think about AIDS by relying, even with the greatest mistrust, on subjectivity (and Derrida has demonstrated that the concepts of historicity and epochality derive from the concept of subjectivity, from the concept itself), it is only because the virus weakens the subjective recuperation of the event, because it loosens and unhinges the "stabilizing arrest" [*arrêt stabilisateur*], which one calls "the subject." We give credence to the subject, we credit it, only after having denied it credit. AIDS not only receives credit through the confession, as Guibert maintains. It decides on creditworthiness itself. However, is not the emergence and epidemic spread of AIDS exactly that event which poses the challenge to think its own im-pertinence? This im-pertinence consists in the impossibility, for the event, of appropriating itself and of belonging to itself. This does not mean, however, that it therefore simply belongs to that which is not event-like. A thinking that concerns itself with AIDS, with the event of its emergence and spread, with contamination and the relation between event and contamination, seems unable to prevent its own contamination, to prevent AIDS.

"The virus (which belongs neither to life nor to death) may *always already* have afflicted and broken into any 'intersubjective' trajectory," Derrida insists in the interview "The Rhetoric of Drugs." At this point in the interview, conducted in the same year as the interview on the subject, Derrida calls AIDS a hitherto "completely unknown" and now "indelible given" [*donnée absolument originale et ineffaçable*], which marks "our time."[2] How should one think the specificity, the originality, the novelty, the event-like dimension of *this* event, if the emergence of AIDS is determined by the fact that it refers back to something that *always already* may have happened, that *always already* has happened, that *always already* has broken into thinking, that always already has been said or spoken by the thinking of this "*always-already*"? Is the emergence of AIDS *the event of the event* and thus that which only happens by giving way to a sort of "retreat into the event" [*Einkehr in das Ereignis*]? What is at stake in the time of this event—of the event—what is at stake in "our time"? Derrida says, "And given its spatial and temporal dimensions, its structure of relays and delays, no human being is ever safe from AIDS. This possibility is thus installed at the heart of the social bond as intersubjectivity. And at the heart of that which would preserve itself as a dual intersubjectivity it inscribes the mortal and indelible trace of the third party—not the third term as the condition of the symbolic and the law, but the third as destructuring structuration of the social bond, as social disconnection (*délaison*) and even as the disconnection of the interruption, of the 'without relation' that can constitute a relation to the other in its alleged normality. The third itself is no longer a third, and the history of this normality more clearly displays its simulacra, almost as if AIDS painted a picture of its exposed anatomy. You may say this is how it's always been, and I believe it. But now, exactly as if it were a painting or a giant movie screen, AIDS provides an available, daily, massive *readability* to that which the canonical discourses . . . had to deny, which in truth they are destined to deny, founded as they are by this very denial" (Derrida [4], pp. 251/211–12). To the degree to which it concerns itself with AIDS, with the emergence and spread of the virus, the thinking of deconstruction, which is a thinking of contagion or of contamination, must approach two questions.

1. If deconstruction still gives credence to historicity, if it trusts in historicity up to a certain point and under certain circumstances—what then does it share with Heidegger, what does it still have in common with Heidegger?

2. If deconstruction recognizes (itself in) AIDS, if AIDS recognizes itself in deconstruction, if deconstruction and AIDS recognize one another—what does such a recognition mean, what does it mean that both deconstruction and AIDS acknowledge each other's existence, that they acknowledge their own existence in the existence of the other?

Ad 1—Deconstruction, Historicity, AIDS. Whoever understands the emergence and epidemic spread of AIDS as a "historical" event—and at the same time emphasizes the impossibility of a discourse based on such an understanding—directs attention to those passages in Heidegger that deal with sickness. What place does the sickness have in the analysis of history and historicity? To begin with, it may be sufficient to point to two paragraphs in which Heidegger mentions and even develops the motif or theme of sickness.

The paragraph in *Being and Time* that delimits the existential analysis of death in order to distinguish it from all other interpretations that have death as their object refers to the phenomenon of being sick and does so in a way entirely in accord with the project of a fundamental ontology. Heidegger actually suggests (Is it a matter of a mere hypothesis?) that we think sickness as existential phenomenon. He mentions sickness at the point he mentions death and adds that the existential understanding of these two phenomena also affects medicine. He does not merely want to claim, however, that physicians who would comprehend the essential and decisive features of the science they practice must obtain an ontological understanding of Dasein and the relationship among Dasein, death, and sickness *in retrospect*. Heidegger's gesture is much more radical, not at all satisfied with a distribution that concedes a certain autonomy to positivist science if only it eventually followed the directives of fundamental ontology: "Medical and biological investigation into 'demising' [into the 'intermediate phenomenon,' which is supposed to be neither a perishing nor a dying—author's note] can obtain results which may even become significant ontologically if the basic orientation for an existential interpretation of death has been made secure. Or must sickness and death in general—even from a medical point of view—be primarily conceived as existential phenomena?" (Heidegger [1], p. 291/247).[3] From whatever viewpoint one considers its symptoms, in the final analysis sickness remains an existential phenomenon, as does death. Perhaps it is important at this point to understand sickness as something that affects Dasein itself, Dasein in its entirety or as a whole; perhaps it is necessary to understand that one cannot think the possibility of a "potentiality for Being-a-whole" [*Ganzseinkönnen*], which is supposed to characterize Dasein, without thinking sickness and "understanding [it] as primarily existential."

In order to attain the primordiality or originality of an ontological ground, on which every possible interpretation of existence is based, the existential analytic must analyze the potentiality-for-Being-a-whole of that being [*Seiendes*] which alone has an understanding of Being [*Sein*]. Heidegger begins by outlining the boundaries that constitute this Being-a-whole and that bestow on it a distinguishable shape (the shape of the incomplete and of that which is yet outstanding) without being able to bestow this shape on it completely. For as soon as the boundaries draw the outlines of this shape, they open it up to a shapeless outside or a shapeless incompleteness; they open it to something that is shapeless because it is still outstanding. Heidegger writes, "As long as Dasein is, there is in every case something still outstanding, which Dasein can be and will be" (p. 276/233). The end of "Being-in-the-world," "Dasein's Being-at-an-end in death," is pertinent because it "belongs to existence," to that existence which is something outstanding, a potentiality-for-Being. Of course, the interpretation of Dasein as something that relates to death as outstanding turns it into something present-at-hand, and Heidegger therefore says that death rather stands before our existence (see p. 294/250). Death belongs to Dasein, to which, however, it cannot be in a simple relationship of "belonging": it "limits and determines in every case whatever totality is possible for Dasein." The phenomenal and ontological understanding of potentiality-for-Being-a-whole thus depends on an existential notion of death. The "existential structure of Being-toward-death" is nothing other than "the ontologically constitutive state of Dasein's potentiality-for-Being-a-whole." If now temporality is "the primordial ontological ground for Dasein's existentiality," if on the basis of a non-vulgar conception of time we can understand why Dasein is fundamentally historical, it becomes clear that the phenomenon of sickness, which Heidegger relates immediately to the phenomenon of death, cannot be understood as long as it is not thought in its connection with the potentiality-for-Being-a-whole of historical Dasein.

In a passage of the transcription of the lecture course that he

dedicated to Schelling in 1936, Heidegger again takes up the motif
or theme of sickness, barely touched upon in *Being and Time* and
only mentioned in the sentence quoted above. Heidegger establishes an essential relationship between disease and existence as a
whole, between the dissolution of the totality in disease and the
overall state or condition of existence, and he does so explicitly.
But as is so often the case in reading the comprehensive, recon-
structive interpretations by means of which Heidegger approaches
thinkers and poets, it is not easy to decide what meaning to ascribe
to this explicit linking of the two. Do we have here a discussion
or explication that concerns only the text to which it refers? Or
does Heidegger also speak in his own name? Maybe the first hypothesis does not exclude the second one: "By way of clarifying
malice Schelling mentions disease. Disease makes itself felt to 'feeling' as something very real, not just as a mere absence of something. When a man is sick, we do say that he 'is not quite all right'
[*daß ihm etwas 'fehle'*] and thus express the sickness merely nega-
tively as a lack. But this: 'Why is he not quite right?' [*'Wo fehlt
es?'*] really means 'What is the matter with him? Something has, so
to speak, gotten loose from the harmony of being healthy and, being on the loose, wants to take over all of existence and dominate
it.' In the case of sickness, there is not just something lacking, but
something wrong [*falsch*]. 'Wrong' not in the sense of something
only incorrect, but in the genuine sense of falsification, distortion,
and reversal. This falsification is at the same time false in the sense
of what is sly. We speak of malignant disease. Disease is not only a
disruption, but a reversal of the *whole existence* which takes over
the *total condition* and dominates it" (Heidegger [6], pp. 143–44/
172–73; my emphasis). An attentive reading of this passage should
begin by relating it to the entire lecture course and would have to
situate its statements within that context. When Heidegger says
that disease is not merely a negative phenomenon, he is in accord
with Schelling, that is, with one of the decisive points in the *Treatise on the Essence of Human Freedom*, namely, with the thought
that evil cannot be considered mere negativity. On several occasions, Heidegger returns to the point that evil is nothing negative

in Schelling's treatise, that its ground is positive. At the same time, an interpretive reading, concerned with details and aimed at a comprehensive reconstruction, would have to mark the relation between the mystical-romantic tradition of the German philosophy of nature and the interpretation of disease that Heidegger elucidates *and* proposes himself. Furthermore, such a reading would have to pay attention to the differences that differentiate Heidegger's use of privative concepts elsewhere. But first and foremost it would have to compare the statements about the falsity of disease with the writings on the question concerning truth. In his lecture course on Parmenides, for example, held in the winter semester of 1942–43, Heidegger examines the etymology of the German word *falsch* [wrong] and enters it into the Greco-Latin-English history of translation, which both reveals and conceals the essence of truth. The series in question consists of the expressions *pseudos*, *falsum*, and *trick*. *Pseudos* is a Greek word that, according to Heidegger, belongs to the essential field of *aletheia*. *Falsum* is a Latin translation that inverts the meaning of *pseudos* by incorporating it into the imperial space of craftiness and cunning, of bringing-to-a-fall. In German, *trick* is a foreign word of Anglo-Saxon descent, a descent that Heidegger points out must not be evaluated as contingent.

Immediately after the passage just quoted, the lecture course on Schelling points to the bond that links sickness and truth. Heidegger attempts to find an explanation for this confusion that interferes with our understanding sickness. Why do we misunderstand the *wrong* to which sickness points as "disruption," as a simple, that is a temporary or partial change, as aberration effected from outside, as interference in the mechanism? If we let ourselves be deceived in thinking about *wrongness*, if we falsify or invert *wrongness* (this is a sort of sickness of the wrong), it is because we persist in representing wrongness according to the logical model of the *negative* proposition. Negation, which "revolts as reversal in evil" and in disease, which manifests itself in both evil and disease as wrongness or reversal, resists comprehension as long as propositions follow this model and remain "simple sentence[s] about a real state of things [*dinglichen Sachverhalt*]" (Heidegger [6], p. 144/173). The expression "a real state of things" implicitly points the reader to Heidegger's lecture *On the Essence of Truth*, which opens with a discussion of the relationship between propositional statement and thing. In order to avoid the confusion that limits us to a merely negative thinking of disease, we must think the disharmony and discord that can be felt in being sick from the point of view of consonance and accord or harmony. That is, there is an originary affirmation and assent without which we have no access to the negation, falsification, and inversion of sickness and of evil: "What replaces the place of harmony and attunement is disharmony, the wrong tone which *enters the whole*. Primordially conceived, affirmation is not just the recognition coming afterward from without of something already existing; it is an assent, a yes harmonizing everything, penetrating and putting it in tune with itself; similarly the no" (ibid.; my emphasis). This similarity, which Heidegger does not describe, is, however, asymmetrical. If "negation is not just rejection of what is objectively present," the reason for this is that "no-saying" is supposed "to place itself in the position of the yes" (ibid.), and by doing so turn the position of the whole that has been understood "primordially enough" (the position of the whole existence, the position of its total condition) into a position that is dissonant and out of tune. Here sickness is perceived as the falsifying, distracting exposure of accord and harmony, as a multiplication of voices to the point of discord and disharmony, as (de-)positing and dismaying dissonance, which destroys "the essential unity of a being as a whole," detaches the "with-and-in-itself" from the "in-tune-with-and-in-itself" and engenders a "reversed unity"—but still a unity, since Heidegger still comprehends negation as position. However, the perverting negation, negation as sickness, is possible only where what is ordered and joined in the "yes" that harmonizes everything is traversed by a difference; it is possible only where the "yes" itself displays an opening, a latitude, a minimal distance, a certain freedom. This latitude, this freedom always already exposes Being-with-and-in-itself to an outside and can neither be reduced to originary affirmation nor to true negation, neither to consonance nor to dissonance, neither to the *unity* of what holds together nor to the *unity* of what turns against it. Rather, this latitude and freedom must be thought as a dis-united "yes/no," which permits the production of both unities; they must be thought as originary Being-not-one or as originary im-pertinence—which necessarily elude the recognition of the "yes" in the "no"—of the attuned totality in its inversion, of disease. It is precisely this structure, that is, the unstable structure of primordial Being-not-one, of pre-primordiality in the primordial, that Heidegger points out after discussing originary affirmation and true negation, at the very moment he returns to Schelling's thoughts about evil and freedom and to the relation of ground to existence. Heidegger underlines the instability that contaminates the origin and makes it possible. Is such thinking still a "philosophy of origin"? "Negation as reversal is thus only and truly possible when ground and existence (both are in themselves ordered in such a way that they relate to each other) become free to move and thus make it possible for the unity to be reversed" (ibid.). Heidegger leaves no doubt that the reversal never touches the unity itself. But perhaps there is not even a unity that could posit itself as unity, since all unity seems to depend on a primordial Being-not-one.

Precisely because of the caution necessary here, we must not reductively label Heidegger's "holistic" understanding of disease as "anti-scientific" or as a strategy of "counterenlightenment." In light of this understanding, how can we respond to the peculiar credence Derrida seems to give the concepts of fundamental ontology and of the thinking of Being? If we want to pave a connection between Heidegger's reflections on sickness[4] and Derrida's remarks about AIDS in order to formalize the feature common to these discourses and transform it into a kind of axiom, perhaps we must venture the following claim: sickness can *become significant* for thought, it can *have a signification*; but it *has a signification*, it *becomes significant* for thought only at the moment it is and must be thought as that which delimits, determines, constitutes, inverts, destructures, deconstructs, a whole or a unity. The sickness of thinking threatens the whole and by no means remains "external" to it. Every time, it is a lethal and consequently historical—or almost historical—sickness. Must we not resort to this axiom to clarify the relation between confession and sickness or disease?

However, is AIDS (still) a disease? And if it is (still) a disease, is it an ancient disease that has been around for a long time, or is it novel, even a novel type of, disease? Since the discovery of the HIV-retrovirus, which has provoked and continues to provoke scientific, legal, institutional, international, disputes, the etiological definition of AIDS has changed: it no longer corresponds to the definition of a syndrome. AIDS is now defined as a "retroviral infectious disease" (Grmek, p. 33/71). As to whether the pandemic infection caused by the virus can be described as a new type of disease, Grmek answers: "It is not a disease in the old sense of the word, inasmuch as the virus is immunopathogenic, that is, it affects the immune system and produces symptoms only through the expedient of opportunistic infection or malignancy. However, AIDS can be partially conceived as a disease in the classical sense inasmuch as the virus can also exert a direct cytopathogenic action, that is, it can directly affect, impede, or destroy certain cells" (p. 109/187). On the other hand, "AIDS is definitely new in its present epidemiological dimension. In the past, biological and social conditions prevented a major outbreak of a retroviral infection transmitted in such a special manner, and especially one that so ruthlessly attacks the immune system. A disastrous epidemic of this type could not have occurred before the mingling of peoples, the liberalization of sexual and social mores, and, above all, before progress in modern medicine had accomplished the control of the majority of serious infectious diseases and introduced intravenous injections and blood transfusion. All this does not necessarily imply that the virus in question is a newborn in the absolute sense, a mutant whose ancestors were never pathogenic" (pp. 109/187–88).

Ad 2—AIDS, Deconstruction, Re-cognition. The emergence and spread of AIDS, Derrida emphasizes repeatedly, is an event that leaves indelible traces and has irreversible effects, and that always holds something of itself in reserve. That we might someday develop a vaccine to control AIDS changes nothing here. The "indestructibility" of that which belongs to the order of events is due precisely to its own destructive force and is not simply opposed to destruction: a singularity or uniqueness (of the event) that is all the more unique because it exposes the singular or unique to contamination, to infection, to generalized immune deficiency. Derrida states, "If I spoke a moment ago of an event and of indestructibility, it is because already, at the dawn of this very new and ever so ancient thing, we know that, even should humanity someday come to control the virus (it will take at least a generation), still, even in the most unconscious symbolic zones, the traumatism has irreversibly affected our experience of desire and of what we blithely call intersubjectivity, the relation to the alter ego, and so forth" (Derrida [4], p. 251/212). A traumatic experience, whose effects one assumes are irreversible, is an experience that precedes any form of memory or recollection. If we reconstruct the "logic" of Derrida's remarks, we will have to say that the emergence and epidemic spread of AIDS destructure a certain organization of society, because they are the cause of a trauma at once novel and immemorial. Time is always the time of AIDS, AIDS time. But this assertion does not preclude the worldwide spread of the virus from being "a historic (historial!) knot or dénouement which is no doubt original" (p. 252/212).

To be sure, the fact that an effective medical strategy to fight AIDS has not (yet) been found should not lead us to recognize in the disease the "economy of death," of which Derrida writes in other contexts, an economy that describes the spacing of writing (see *Of Grammatology*), and that produces itself as or in *différance* (*Différance*). But perhaps it is easier to understand why in Derrida's texts the HIV infection is assigned such prominence if we take into consideration its specificity. The "classic model of infection," as Grmek explains, "places the invading microbe in frank opposition to the cell." But HIV, this retrovirus, acts as a parasite that just inscribes itself in "the very heart of the host's control center," which defines the cell, *without opposing it.* "Integrated like this into the cell genome, the virus temporarily loses its individuality and can remain latent for a number of years. During this period, the cell appears to be normal and the virus seems to disappear. Its essential part is hidden in the form of a so-called provirus, a piece of viral DNA attached to the host DNA. In this state, the virus is invulnerable to drugs; it can be destroyed only by killing the cell. The proviral DNA *may be silent,* but it is still 'alive' because it is transmitted to every daughter cell after each cellular division" (Grmek, pp. 78/140–42; my emphasis). The transition to a state that is called HIV-positive—and bears the French name *séroconversion*: transformation, inversion, conversion of the blood—happens only later, when another infection activates the lymphocyte infected with HIV. "The provirus can 'wake up.' It takes over the enzymes and ribosomes of the host cell, inducing them to make viruses" (ibid.). Is not deconstruction also a kind of virus that one day "wakes up"? If no system, no concept, no thought, no culture, no nature, is exempt from deconstruction, if there is always already deconstruction, then the intervention of a deconstruction that can be called by its ("im-proper") name is no less an event. As an event that receives a name, deconstruction happens at a specific point in time, *today*; hence the semblance of stability offered, for a longer or shorter period of time, by that which is untouched and simultaneously infected. Does deconstruction, then, recognize itself in the (mirror) image that the wide screen of AIDS holds up to it? Does it decipher itself as the image projected on this "mirroring screen"? A peculiar and confusing speculation, a non-speculative speculation: the recognition implied by the "massive legibility" allegedly produced by the emergence and spread of AIDS cannot be a *recognizing oneself that produces an identity*, but is recognizable enough to permit us to speak of a *recognition of deconstruction*. It is as if deconstruction would recognize and acknowledge AIDS because it recognizes itself in it. The time of AIDS, AIDS time, is a caesura in time. It is the untimely moment when deconstruction continues deconstructing *and* interrupts "itself."

Because deconstructive "work" (Derrida [5], p. 390) is not the work or the labor of the concept, the recognition of deconstruction differs from self-recognition, from a recognition that produces an identity. Deconstruction cannot relate to itself as a subject does. But after reading the interview "The Rhetoric of Drugs," after reading what is said there about the event "of our time," one is undoubtedly inclined to assume that Derrida says nothing about AIDS he would not have said about deconstruction. Admittedly, it would probably be facile to suspect the gesture of recognition of being nothing more than a gesture of appropriation—a gesture of appropriating that which is recognized or recognizes itself. Nevertheless, such a suspicion would not be groundless. Why? This question allows us, perhaps, to touch on the paradox of a thought that does not recollect or assemble itself in an identity of the identical and the non-identical. For if thought always has the task of thinking that which cannot be reduced to itself, if we think only when we pursue this task, then there is no thinking that does not distinguish itself as something excessive and that does not turn out to be essentially im-pertinent. When Adorno, for example, declares that the truth of psychoanalysis depends on its exaggerations, when he defines philosophy as the thinking of that which thought itself is not, he clearly points to this constitutive excess of all thinking. For a thinking that cannot absorb its own excess and thus make it commensurable, for a thinking that does not sublate its im-pertinence, recognition cannot designate a point at which the subject relates itself to itself, defining itself as subject and appropriating all its elements with no excess outstanding. But the reason recognition always exposes itself to the suspicion of being a (re)appropriation is that it inescapably implies a certain *self*-recognition, a certain recognizing *oneself.* Thus it could almost be said that a thinking not-at-one with AIDS, that wishes to fight AIDS, requires a supplement of im-pertinence. But in what does the im-pertinence of thought consist when it strives to think AIDS and its consequences, when it is required in the process to *recognize itself in a Being-not-one that is its "own" Being-not-one?* That is the question of deconstruction, and of any thinking that measures up to it in the time of AIDS, in AIDS time.

Afterword

Those with whom I will have thought and talked about AIDS, in no particular order: with J., who explained to me why in his confessions he talks about a Jew in New York who is ill with AIDS; I try to recall his explanation. With H., who thinks that only a strictly positivist method is justified when one thinks and talks about AIDS. With J.-L., who writes me that his survival depends on the controlled inducement of an immune deficiency. With W., who calls the epidemic a produced death. With C., who wonders about the pathos of distance with which I allegedly wrote my essay. With G., who defends himself against intimidation, doubts the results of research, and is met with incomprehension because he does not unequivocally advise safer sex. With S., who encourages me to express anger in an undisguised and blunt manner. With T., who pretends to be interested in my work and describes his library full of literature about AIDS; he wants to give me hundreds of books and insists that I call him; eventually, he brings not a single book along. With G., who makes clear to me that the desire to have a fate amounts to the desire for a narratable life history; she tells me the story of a man who wanders around desperately and attempts in vain for an entire night to extinguish a fire that is destroying all he has; the following morning he recognizes that the tracks he left in the sand come together as the lines of an image. With T., who would like to combine his insights with new forms of activism. With you, day and night and never.

The present essay represents the substantially enlarged, altered, and corrected version of a talk I wrote in French and gave in the seminar of Jacques Derrida (March 1991). In an English translation by Andrew Hewitt, I repeated this talk at a conference in Buffalo (October 1991). The French text, bearing the title *Ce qu'on aura pu dire du sida: Quelques remarques dans le désordre*, appeared in the journal *Po&sie* (Paris, December 1991), the English translation—*What Will Have Been Said About AIDS: Some Remarks in Disorder*—in *Public* (Toronto, Winter 1992). I especially want to thank Werner Hamacher and Thomas Keenan; I also would like to thank Stephen Andrews, Adam Rolston, and Brian Weil, as well as Petra Eggers, who took the book under her care. Without her confidence in the project, the book would not have been written. I am grateful to Conrad Scott-Curtis and Peter Gilgen, the translators of *At Odds with AIDS*. Their philosophical insight, their linguistic skills, and their endurance have contributed a great deal to making this book accessible to American and English readers.

The general thesis of the essay is: *Only an existence that is a primordial non-belonging, an im-pertinence that precedes every belonging, can measure up to AIDS—to the uncertainty of all boundaries—and meet the challenge posed by the epidemic.* I leave it to the reader to decide whether the orientation of extensive passages to the relation between (male) homosexuality and AIDS proves to be relevant for this thesis, whether this orientation predetermines the whole essay in a decisive way and thus itself contradicts the notion of im-pertinence. However, I do not know exactly what it means to talk about such an orientation, since the current explanations and justifications of the concept of (male) homosexuality leave me increasingly perplexed.

A.G.D.
San Francisco, November 1992

Reference Matter

Notes

Chapter 1

1. With the distinction between "not-at-one" and "not-one," we attempt to translate García Düttmann's use of *uneins* and *un-eins* as distinct concepts. For a more complete discussion of these concepts and our rendering of them in English, see the "Translators' Note" preceding the main text—translators' note.

2. Heidegger's existential analytic emphasizes the simultaneity of certainty and indefiniteness as distinguishing Dasein's relationship to death "in general." Perhaps it is not only a threat to Dasein—a threat "kept open" by anxiety—that lies in this simultaneity, but also the hope without which Dasein could not "cling tenaciously to" the possibility of existence it has seized upon. If thus death does *not* "constitute the entirety of existence" (Adorno [1], p. 369/360)—Adorno asserts this against Heidegger with polemical intent—this is the case because Dasein is Being-towards-death and because finitude defines its condition. Heidegger says that hope "must be analyzed in much the same way as fear" and that it is ontologically possible only "if Dasein has an ecstatic-temporal relation to the thrown ground of itself" (Heidegger [1], pp. 395–96/345). Hope is grounded in the future of "anticipating death" [*Vorlaufen in den Tod*] precisely to the degree to which the temporal mode of this relation has the character of "having been": "Only so far as it is futural can Dasein *be* as having been. The character of 'having been' arises, in a certain way, from the future" (p. 373/326).

3. Wherever a unity is supposed to be established, it is a matter of a

tying back into, even when this unity is not lamented as lost, but promised as still outstanding: if there is a unity at all—and precisely that is in question—then it must *per definitionem* precede Being-not-one; whether as past or yet to come, unity must take priority over it.

4. The paperback edition of the novel *Le très-haut,* which Maurice Blanchot first published in 1948 and revised in 1975, appeared in 1988— 40 years after the first edition—with a jacket blurb specifically written for the newest edition. The blurb, presumably authorized if not written by the author, contains a paragraph starting with the sentences, "The highest, that which is perfect can only be its own negation. In a perfect society, in which the plague breaks out and the plague victims become the only rebels, in which AIDS threatens the highest law. . . . " Does AIDS accede to the symbolic inheritance of the plague?

5. One should be suspicious of all those edifying, apologetic, and appeasing discourses that interpret the certainty of an almost definite death as *memento mori,* as an admonition that reminds us of finitude. Seneca's *De brevitate vitae* makes clear that the remembrance of finitude is not at all incompatible with the idea of a unity of life. The (virtual) merging of the certainty and definiteness of death, however, does not leave this idea untouched: one must not immediately equate dying "before one's time" with finitude. Life is experienced as short, writes Seneca, only by the person who does not understand how to live, that is to say who does not fashion every day as if it were his last. Therefore, everything depends on the way we treat life—on whether we succeed in producing a unity of life that collects the past, present, and future in a single time. Only someone who does not die before his time, who withdraws and masters time, who does not want to begin to live only at the instant the life force leaves his body, who is capable of administering the life capital that is entrusted to him for an indeterminate period. The sage alone dies at the right time; he who dies at the right time is a sage: "But for those whose life is passed remote from all business, why should it not be ample? None of it is assigned to another, none of it is scattered in this direction or that, none of it is committed to Fortune, none of it perishes from neglect, none is subtracted by wasteful giving, none of it is unused; the whole of it, so to speak, yields income. And so, however small the amount of it, it is abundantly sufficient, and therefore, whenever his last day shall come, the wise man will not hesitate to go to meet death with a steady step" (Seneca, p. 321). Dying "before one's time," toward which the existence of HIV-positive people and those with AIDS seems di-

rected, is thus not just evidence of finitude. Rather, it is evidence of the failure of the attempt to sublate the shortness of life in a unity of life. The difficulties that accompany this attempt perhaps become obvious in Seneca's treatise where he says that one needs an entire life to learn living and dying—to become a sage. How short and how long is a life that only at its end opens up the possibility of its own unification?

For Montaigne, the evaluation of another depends on his dying. The last day of life is at the same time the first, because life receives its meaning from that day: "In judging the life of another, I always observe how it ended" (Montaigne, p. 55/125). In principle, though, there is always only a last day of life. Every day can be the day of reckoning. "It is uncertain where death awaits us; let us await it everywhere" (p. 60/132). If we must expect death everywhere and at each point in time, if we always live our last day, it is because we incessantly flee ourselves, because we die while living ("pendant la vie vous estes mourant") and because one never dies before one's time ("nul ne meurt avant son heure"). Wherever the certainty and indefiniteness of death belong together essentially, one cannot die before one's time, and the thought that one dies before one's time actually cannot arise. But is it possible to expect that which one experiences only once, and which therefore precisely cannot be experienced? Montaigne emphasizes the uniqueness of death in order to deprive it of its terror. Here, everything is inverted, but Montaigne does not reflect on this inversion. Precisely the uniqueness and irreversibility of death render it frightful. By the same token, one could claim that the impossibility of experiencing death—its singularity—frustrates any possibility of expecting its arrival, whereas quite possibly nothing other can be expected than that which one has not always already anticipated, that which does not inevitably imply a jump out of the possible and a foothold in the actual. If the utility of life (*utilité du vivre*) is not measured in terms of space, that is, of length and duration, but in terms of use of life (*usage*)—a thought that again seems to lead back to Seneca— then this use is split by the expectation of that which cannot be experienced but which defines our lives. Now, what use of life can somebody make who knows he will probably die "before his time," somebody for whom the certainty and definiteness of death thus tend to coincide? What does "use" mean in this case? Jean Starobinski, who stresses the passages in the *Essais* in which Montaigne denies the privileged truth of the last hour, guides our view to another paradox: it is not only its incommensurability but also its ubiquity that undermines and destroys death (Starobinski, pp. 75–76/96–98). Heidegger's formulation of death as the possibility of the impossibility of Dasein draws the consequence from this paradox, as it were. Death can be thought only as an aporia: death is constitutive of Dasein and is *at the same time* its absolute limit; it is the one *because* it is the other.

6. Enlightenment does not distinguish between risk and its opposite, but "between the necessary restriction of risk and the idea that one could eliminate risk, which is an illusion" (Dannecker [2]).

7. Gregg Araki's movie, *The Living End* (1992), shows a type of challenge that is not a reaffirmation, but rather the unmediated result of the state of emergency brought about by the certainty and definiteness of death. This state of emergency removes the individual from valid normative relations: the absolute autonomy produced by the heteronomy of the fatal infection can turn the individual into a figure of justice that appears as violence and that no justification can overtake. Jochen Hick's film *Via Appia*, a TV movie with little ambition, and perhaps precisely because of that appropriate to its subject, does not depict the transformation of the everyday into a state of emergency caused by AIDS. Rather, it shows the integration of the disease into the everyday, into the life of an airline steward, who during a vacation in Rio de Janeiro is looking for a hustler who cannot be found. This life is uneventful and determined by inconspicuous, never spectacularly disruptive changes; even a mutilation scene does not come across as something extraordinary. The movie *Poison*, shot by Todd Haines in 1991, is a story that can be understood as the transposition of the subject of the uncontrollable, massive epidemic into the genre of the science-fiction B-picture of the 1950's.

8. Could one not even, with reference to a passage from the *Genealogy of Morals*, describe the retrospective view as that which Nietzsche calls "a deadening of pain by means of affects"? "The suffering are one and all dreadfully eager and inventive in discovering occasions for painful affects; . . . they scour the entrails of their past and present for obscure and questionable occurrences that offer them the opportunity to revel in tormenting suspicions and to intoxicate themselves with the poison of their own malice; . . . they tear open their oldest wounds, they bleed from long-healed scars" (Nietzsche [2], pp. 127–28/374–75).

9. The truth at stake here is perhaps the one Jacques Derrida captures in a passage on Augustine's *Confessions*: "Making *truth* has no doubt

nothing to do with what you call truth, for in order to confess it is not enough to *bring to knowledge*, to make *known what is*, for example to *inform* you that I have brought death, that I have killed, betrayed, blasphemed, perjured, it is not enough that I *present myself* to God or to you, for truth, the presentation of what is or what I am, either by revelation or by adequate judgment, has never given rise to avowal, to true avowal: the *essential* truth of avowal has nothing to do with truth . . . " (Derrida [1], p. 48/49). Consequently, AIDS is not *my* AIDS because I announce that the virus is in *my* body but because I decide to declare allegiance to AIDS and to come to myself in this way. In this connection, the mark "AIDS" functions as the name of the decision, of the resolution by means of which one declares allegiance to oneself and produces the truth—in an article, in front of witnesses, in the face of the Other.

The distinction between a confession that refers to an empirical referent, the adequacy of which can therefore be tested, and a confession that cannot be pinned down empirically because it expresses a feeling—the "inner truth" of which the referent is the external complement—must be considered problematic from such a perspective. This distinction is quoted, for example, at the beginning of Paul de Man's essay on Rousseau's *Confessions*: "To confess is to overcome guilt and shame in the name of truth: it is an epistemological use of language in which ethical values of good and evil are superseded by values of truth and falsehood. . . . What Rousseau is saying then, when he insists on '*sentiment intérieur*,' is that confessional language can be considered under a double epistemological perspective: it functions as a verifiable referential cognition, but it also functions as a statement whose reliability cannot be verified by empirical means. The convergence of the two modes is not a priori given, and it is because of the possibility of the discrepancy between them that the possibility of excuse arises" (de Man, pp. 279 and 281). Confessed AIDS is never an external, complexly structured referent, even if such reference—the possibility of medical verification—incites the confession. In regard to the production of truth that happens in or as confession, "inner feeling" is itself a formulation that perhaps refers too strongly to the (sentimental) subject, at least if one abstracts from the historical context of confessions.

10. AIDS is assigned this function as a paradigm of "modernity" probably also because of a specific comparison. For in one passage Guibert compares his wasted, sick body with the body of a person deported

to Auschwitz. Questionable comparison: "This shrunken body . . . I discovered every morning, an Auschwitzian exhibit in the full-length bathroom mirror. . . . Some days I get the feeling he'll make it, because people did come back from Auschwitz . . . " (Guibert [2], pp. 6–7/14–15).

In the final analysis, such analogies can have disastrous consequences. They pave the way for a review that was printed after Guibert's death and that focuses on his book *Cytomégalovirus* (1992). This book is a description, in diary form, of a stay in the hospital before the author's final admission to it. The book's publication is legitimized by the reviewer with the remark that it is a unique document, a document of the "mysterious black source that currently gives its shape to mankind, thus helping it to find again the great lost law" (Christian Charrière, "Hervé Guibert: Pages from the Death Struggle," see *Le Figaro Littéraire* of Feb. 3, 1992). Jean-Luc Nancy, in his text "The Great Law," analyzes and denounces the ideologically reactionary implications of the review: "We are offered the model of a nomodicy; as a theodicy justifies God in and on the basis of his whole creation, including evil, the nomodicy justifies AIDS and bad literature to the degree that they return us to the right path, the path of healthy art and healthy sex" (p. 46).

11. "Some become too old even for their truths and victories: a toothless mouth no longer has the right to every truth." This sentence, for which Heidegger gives no reference (Heidegger [1], pp. 306/262), can be found in *Zarathustra*, more precisely, in the section "On Free Death" that deals with death *at the right time*, and thereby with life lived *at the right time*: "Many die too late, and a few die too early. The doctrine still sounds strange: 'Die at the right time!' Die at the right time—thus teaches Zarathustra. Of course, how could those who never live at the right time die at the right time? Would that they had never been born! . . . Free to die and free in death, able to say a holy No when the time for Yes has passed: thus he knows how to die and to live" (Nietzsche [1], pp. 183–85/93–95).

12. In fundamental ontology, certainty can be brought back to the "certainty of Dasein," which is the certainty of indefinite death. Because Dasein can seize its "ownmost possibility," through which it discloses its "ownmost potentiality-for-Being," only as a Dasein that anticipates death, every other understanding of the certainty must remain a subordinate, derivative understanding. The certainty of the "event which one encounters in one's own environment," the empirical certainty, the "apodictic" certainty that "we reach in certain domains of theoretical

knowledge," all presuppose the "certainty of Dasein." The fundamental certainty, without which we would not even know what certainty can be, is the certainty accompanied by indefiniteness: only if we think the link between indefiniteness and certainty will we gain access to this certainty and no longer cover it up. Thus, certainty originally is no concept of theory, but must be connected to the "attunement [*Gestimmtheit*] [of a] state-of-mind," to anxiety, which holds open a threat: Dasein is threatened by a death both certain and indefinite. Does not Wittgenstein also point to the nexus between certainty and mood [*Stimmung*] when he remarks that certainty is "*as it were* a tone of voice in which one declares how things are"? (Wittgenstein [1], p. 6) But how does the "certainty of Dasein" relate to subjectivity—to the history of truth and to the truth of history in the "course" of which the Cartesian *certitudo* inaugurated modernity? "Because truth now means the assuredness of presentation-to [*Zustellung*], or *certainty*, and because Being means representedness in the sense of such certainty, man, in accordance with his role in foundational representation, becomes the subject in a distinctive sense," writes Heidegger in a passage on Descartes's *cogito sum* contained in his 1940 lectures on "European Nihilism" (Heidegger [2], p. 117/166).

13. What is more definite than this "unmediated" moment, without which one could not disclose temporality, and which perhaps is not even "temporal," not even a moment, even if the moment forever keeps itself in resoluteness, in "anticipation" of the (im)possibility of death? Can one say in the expectation of this "unmediated" moment, in an expectation that can barely be experienced, in an expectation that is not an expectation: "not right away"? What is more indefinite than this "unmediated" moment? Does not its "immediacy" transform it into an "abstract" moment, into an "unmediated" moment that, in its very "immediacy," is always already "past" and still "outstanding"—so that one can only say, "not right away"?

14. Does the irreducibility of such tensions invoke the type of criticism of fundamental ontology that accuses it of "thinning out" concepts "drawn from life" into "a prioris of existence" (Schweppenhäuser, p. 60)?

15. In this context, the (phenomenological) "as such" must of course be subjected to that "essential transformation" Derrida speaks of when investigating the "paradoxical representation of the unrepresentable as such" (Derrida [2], p. 85). This transformation is required by Being-not-one, which cannot just show or present itself as a phenomenon.

16. Against all positivists, who shy away from any justification, with-

out however being able to explain why one talks so much about AIDS, one could cite a proposition that situates itself on a limit: The facts that amount to the world are in need of "the non-factual, so that they can be recognized from it" (Ingeborg Bachmann).

Chapter 2

1. One could argue against the first hypothesis that it does not confront AIDS and therefore, at bottom, does not take a position. It is a critical hypothesis because it not only relativizes the event-like character of the epidemic but, in the final analysis, also denies it. Perhaps one takes a position only if one recognizes the incursion of the new, if one exposes oneself to the event-like, which evades any complete identification that could recognize it, and, up to a certain degree at least, paralyzes distinguishing and deciding, the business of critique. On the other hand, it seems equally possible to counter the second hypothesis with the argument that it prevents taking a position and does not itself confront the AIDS epidemic. Blind agreement—unreflective acceptance of that which gives only the semblance of novelty and rupture, of an unbridgeable discontinuity, of an event—already forgoes the capacity of critical scrutiny to draw distinctions and make decisions, and is incapable of taking a position, of confrontation. In a certain way, therefore, the two (originally incompatible) hypotheses complement each other: the space they create is not so much divided as homogeneous.

2. The *Petit Robert* contains the word "trick": " *TRICK ou TRIC; mot anglais, proprem. 'ruse, stratagème,' du norm. 'trikier' (voir 'tricher'). Jeu— Au whist, au bridge, la septième levée, qui est la première (après le 'devoir') à compter un point. Hom.: 'trique'* "; if one looks up *trique*, one reads the following: "*gros bâton, et specialt. bâton utilisé come arme pour frapper.*" If one looks up " *triquer*" in *Harrap's French and English Dictionary of Slang and Colloquialisms* (London, 1980), one finds a cross-reference to "*bander*" [being horny, having an erection]; in English, of course, "a trick" is quick intercourse with a prostitute.

3. A transformation is made apparent here that cannot just be ascribed to the fact that every book is already testimony, even if this transformation is unthinkable without such immediate testimony. Because of this transformation, the provisional character of the change, the "for the time being" of which Camus speaks and which expresses a hope is itself provisional, is itself, as it were, "for the time being."

4. The word "impertinent," which is usually used to signify an un-

due rebellion against authority, originates in legal discourse, where it means "not belonging to the matter at hand," "irrelevant," "off the point"; it derives from the late Latin "*im-pertinens*": "not belonging to (the matter at hand)." Perhaps one could translate "im-pertinent" with "im-proper" and point, by means of the spelling, to its original meaning: "im-proper" is that which does not belong where it is.

5. After having distinguished between the dogmatic and the skeptical step "in matters of pure reason," Kant speaks of a third step that must be taken in order to secure a "dwelling-place for permanent settlement": "namely, to subject to examination, not the facts of reason, but reason itself, in the whole extent of its powers, and as regards its aptitude for pure *a priori* modes of knowledge. This is not the censorship but the *criticism* of reason, whereby not its present *bounds* but its determinate [and necessary] *limits*, not its ignorance on this or that point but its ignorance in regard to all possible questions of a certain kind, are demonstrated from principles, and not merely arrived at by way of conjecture. Skepticism is thus a resting-place for human reason, where it can reflect upon its dogmatic wanderings and make survey of the region in which it finds itself, so that for the future it may be able to choose its path with more certainty. But there is no dwelling-place for permanent settlement. Such can be obtained only through perfect certainty in our knowledge, alike of the objects themselves and of the limits within which all our knowledge of objects is enclosed" (Kant [2], p. 607/695 [B 789]).

6. The paradox of a limit between a phenomenal and a noumenal *space* is of course that the limit is itself in need of yet another limit: "Space has no limits that would separate it from another space and further from a non-space. If space had such a limit, this limit would be drawn in and against a space, which in its turn would have to have such a limit, which would also have to run in a space, and so on" (Hamacher, p. 40).

7. "Mathematics refers to appearances only, and what cannot be an object of sensuous intuition, such as the concepts of metaphysics and of morals, lies entirely without its sphere; it can never lead to them, but neither does it require them" (Kant [1], pp. 101/352–53).

8. A decisive sentence in the *Tractatus* can be understood as referring to Kant's concept of the limit: "The philosophical I is not the man, not the human body or the human soul of which psychology treats, but the metaphysical subject, the limit—not a part of the world" (Wittgenstein [2], p. 153 [5.641]). At the limits of language, which are the limits of the

world of the subject, and between saying and showing, between saying
and indicating [*Zeigen*], a proposition about the limit is formulated. It is
not certain that this proposition can be formulated and uttered clearly,
since "the subject does not belong to the world but . . . is a limit of the
world" (p. 151 [5.632]). Is it an elementary proposition? Probably not: elementary propositions are simple and affirm the existence of facts, that
is, the configuration of stable and simple objects, the totality of which
is called a world. All the difficulties resulting from the peculiar and necessary im-pertinence of the concept of the limit (these difficulties can be
recognized in Kant's thought) seem to reappear in this context—in a
context determined by the attempt to "delimit the unthinkable from the
inside by means of the thinkable." Strictly speaking, Heidegger, too, develops a philosophy of the limit (transcendental philosophy is nothing
else) when he sets out to think an existing transcendence: " 'Dasein transcends' means that it is in the essence of its Being world-producing [*welt-
bildend*], in the sense that it lets world happen and through the world
provides itself with an originary view (image [*Bild*]) which does not
grasp explicitly, yet serves as a model [*Vorbild*] for all manifest beings,
Dasein included" (Heidegger [3], p. 89/158). It cannot be a coincidence
that Heidegger here chooses the same conceptual language he uses in
Kant and the Problem of Metaphysics. The passage just quoted can be
found in his lecture *The Essence of Reasons* [*Vom Wesen des Grundes*],
which begins with an examination of Kant's concept of world.

9. It seems that Heidegger belongs precisely to this tradition, if one
can believe the copy of lecture notes that Víctor Farías published for the
first time. The incomplete copy is a manuscript that was found in papers left by Helene Weiss. Copied "by an unknown female," these were
the lecture notes of a course on logic Heidegger taught in the summer semester of 1934. "If we take up the question of the essence of History,
there is the objection that our claim—that History is the distinguishing
feature of the human—is arbitrary. Negroes are also human beings, and
have no history. And there is also a history of animals, plants, which is
thousands of years old, and probably older than the entire history of human beings. . . . Nature also has its history. But then the Negroes also
have history. Or does nature, after all, have no history? Although nature
can enter the past as vanishing, not everything that vanishes enters history" (Heidegger/Weiss, pp. 38 and 40). If now "the being-sick of the
human" is a "historical happening of the human" (p. 100), one must ask
oneself whether those human beings Heidegger calls "Negroes" and who

cannot even form "peoples," because they must remain without "space and soil," can know diseases. Is AIDS as an epidemic which spreads among the historical peoples without leaving the delimiting concepts of space, soil, people, history untouched, a "being-sick" that indicates the complete nihilism of history? From the point of view of this question and the Janus-headed logic of nihilism that Heidegger explicates, one would have to say that AIDS is both at the same time: a nihilistic opening of history to that which has no history *and* the result of history itself as nihilism; the worst not-being-sick *and* the greatest being-sick, the being-sick that can hardly be distinguished any longer from not-being-sick, that undergoes the most extreme test, and precisely for that reason is at stake in its entirety. The question that must be raised at this point concerns the limit, the Being-not-one of the disease, the im-pertinence of historical happening, of the people, of space, of soil, etc.

10. "World history in general is thus the unfolding of Spirit in time, *as* nature is the unfolding of the Idea in space" (Hegel [1a], 75/96–97; my emphasis). This "analogy" becomes twisted, because time, on the other hand, is the truth of space.

11. "Possibly the sheer concentration of gay people in San Francisco had no parallel in history" (FitzGerald, p. 27).

12. Obviously, one can draw parallels between the "ritualization of safer sex" and attempts, undertaken in North America with idiosyncratic touchiness and puritanic obsession, to free language from its ideological constructions of domination. The aim of such a liberation is the creation of a politically value-neutral, universal rhetoric, which in fact consists of euphemisms—a *safer language* of purity. In both cases, the objective function of the purification is the function of control and counter-control. With the intention of conducting a critique of ideology, one ultimately works into the hands of the state. Not coincidentally, submitting the "private" spheres of human life to the state and its control is one of the unfortunate consequences that accompany the necessity of behavior oriented toward safer sex. It does not matter what measures the apparatus of the state takes in each case—the apparatus that administrates death by providing and withdrawing necessary resources. *The condom is the police; the condom is the state.* In the linguistic purification campaign, time and again, the evil spirit [*Ungeist*] of the equivocal manifests itself, thwarting, for example, the "liberation of the sexus from its juridical impositions" (Adorno [2], p. 59) in the name of egalitarian demands. Those who speak the new universal language are the already hardened figures of

an advertisement in the New York subway that propagates safer sex and addresses a specific group, Hispanics. On the posters, we see Marisol, a woman who is left by her boyfriend Julio because she refuses to sleep with him without using a condom. She justifies her refusal with the words "I love you, but not enough to die for you." No recycled celebration of romantic *Liebestod* and blurring of differences in the service of a discriminating difference are necessary in order to recognize that with the proclaimed primacy of self-preservation the police establish themselves everywhere. One's own concern and the other's concern for health, on which life depends, poisons all relationships, as justified as the concerns may be and as much as they may express friendship and love.

13. Not everybody belongs to such a community. But who does not belong to it, who is not directly or indirectly affected by AIDS? Shortly before the premiere of the second part of his hit play on AIDS and American society in the 1980's, *Angels in America,* Tony Kushner had a "confessional account" printed in the pages of the *New York Times.* Kushner turns against the myth of the individual he discovers in the United States; the author is not an individual but belongs, with his work, to a collective: "From such nets of souls societies, the social world, human life spring. And also plays" (*New York Times,* Nov. 21, 1993, sec. 2, p. 31). The question the reader must ask is whether here one myth is not replaced by another and whether there is not a strict symmetry between the exaltation of individualism and the recourse to "community." In any case, both the individual and the community are meant to secure an identity and to function as its irreducible bearer.

14. In the pamphlet *ACT UP: The AIDS War and Activism,* George M. Carter points out some successes of the group: "Life-saving information is continually distributed as the latest treatments are monitored. New studies of alternative drugs have been initiated due to efforts by ACT UP. Government officials and media have been forced to recognize and at least begin to address specific AIDS issues. Pharmaceutical companies and the insurance industry have been brought into sharp relief as inefficient and wasteful organizations, which are designed to maximize profits with little or no concern for the effect on people's lives" (Carter, p. 1).

15. Perhaps this testing turns out to be a testing only because it is triggered by an experience of shock that disrupts notions of social identity and identification: "As the infected population grew, it became clear that gay men were everywhere—in politics, in Congress, on Wall Street, in

Hollywood, in far-right organizations. In many cases, they were silent and invisible—unlike women and racial minorities. Part of the shock of AIDS was thus the shock of identity" (Treichler [2], p. 200).

16. In a conversation about the AIDS crisis, activist Gregg Bordowitz states that one thinks about this crisis in a way that generates "at once too little knowledge and too much knowledge" (Caruth and Keenan, p. 553). Is this imbalance of knowledge not also the im-pertinence of that which ought to be known and brought to consciousness? Can a primordially im-pertinent existence, which measures itself against this im-pertinence, produce other forms of knowledge; can it produce *forms* of knowledge at all?

Chapter 3

1. The personification of the threat, its stylization as an enemy, is a kind of demagoguery. It can be found not only in openly reactionary and demagogic discourse but also in uplifting, well-meant speech, where it is perhaps all the more dangerous. An example of this is an essay by Antoine Lion, chairman of the society Christians and AIDS (*Chrétiens et Sida*). Here, personification serves the aim pursued by all apologists for the Church who are afflicted with bad conscience: in the final analysis, they are always concerned with a recuperating rationalization of AIDS. Of course, this aim, this strategy, is pursued in a way that gives an impression of broad-mindedness, avoiding any hint of duplicity. Such apologists speak only in their own name and would not want to impose their belief on others. They even show understanding for the doubts of the nonbeliever and in principle respect atheistic positions. They secure general acclaim with measured self-criticism—perhaps the Church has not behaved as one might have been entitled to expect—and with claims couched in the terms of political sermons: one fights so that the social consequences of the AIDS pandemic do not mock and disparage the "unfathomable dignity of each human being" (Lion, p. 175). In the pseudo-poetic tirade that introduces Lion's essay, the virus is transformed into a "black" or "dark visitor" [*un noir visiteur*], who appears suddenly and can no longer be evicted from the premises. "We have to live with him" (p. 170)—with the plague? This visitor attacks randomly. Few can feel secure from him. The philosophical discourse that speaks of nihilism as a guest is recalled in such an image, even if pseudo-tolerance is exhibited and the current epoch is never called nihilistic; the image serves the authoritarian character as a means of suggesting conspiracies

and fanning the flames of paranoia. The more invisible the enemy, the more perverse and cunning, the more dangerous and omnipresent he is. Naturally, this visitor is the devil. He lurks everywhere, even—or rather, precisely—in writing (the four letters of the brand AIDS are the letters of death and condemnation), and he presses hard the upstanding who fight him. Lament and regret, language of the crusades and deeds of war, language of invocation and exorcism, language of the preacher, of a lion's mane wildly thrown off, of rolling eyes, of the index finger raised in warning and accusation, of deictic concretion ("this," "these")—syntax of accumulated adjectives and infinite enumerations, the fascination of which lies precisely in the lack of the copula: one understands the matter at hand, and it is not necessary to point it out specifically by formulating a proposition of the kind "S is P." Can such a discourse be lifted from its hinges by assimilation and exaggeration? Lion murmurs: "He—it, this word, four perilous letters; this micro-organism whose perversity seems devilish, who uses amazing cunning to beat the attacks led against him, striking them powerless, whose surprising complexity leads astray even the assault of a research community that has no equal in history" (ibid.). In order to resist the devilish visitor, in the midst of the fight that disarms even science, Lion appeals to the spiritual resources of humankind: the "night," Being-not-one with AIDS, is in truth "a reserve of power, meaning, and light"; the fight against AIDS a "spiritual quest"; the suffering of people with AIDS typological, an *imitatio Christi*. The faithful, thus provided with a meaning, ought to place their "reserve of meaning" at the disposal of those who are searching for one. Meaning is thus the commodity of proselytism. Of course, the humble Lion can only speak in his own name: "Often one has to be silent at first" (p. 173). And while one writes all of this, one is "perhaps expected elsewhere" (p. 176). In hell, no doubt.

2. The authors give a tentative name to the "abstract, faceless idea": the name of that which is called "nature" in Sade. Blanchot analyzes the complex use Sade makes of the concept of nature, a use that shows how Sade draws the most radical consequences from Enlightenment philosophy: "In Sade's system, this spirit of destruction is identified with nature. . . . 'Nature' is one of the words that Sade, like so many writers of his time, is all too fond of. It is in the name of nature that he carries out the struggle against God and all God represents, in particular morals. . . . For him, this nature is first and foremost universal life, and for hundreds

of pages his philosophy consists of repeating that the immoral instincts are good since they are natural facts and since nature is the original and final authority. . . . But, then, bothered by the equal value he must ascribe to the virtuous instincts, he tries to establish a new scale of values with crime at its pinnacle. His main argument is that crime is more adequate to the spirit of nature because it is movement, that is, life. Nature, which wants to create, says Sade, is in need of crime that destroys. . . . However, because he always talks of nature, because he always finds himself facing this unavoidable and sovereign reference, the man de Sade becomes increasingly irritated, and his hatred soon makes nature so unbearable for him he covers her with curses and negations: '*Yes, my friend, yes: I abhor nature.*' This revolt has two deep motifs. On the one hand, it seems intolerable to Sade that the unparalleled power of destruction, which he represents, has no purpose other than empowering nature to create. On the other hand, to the degree to which he is himself part of nature, he feels that nature escapes his negation and that the more he rages against her and the better he serves her, the more he negates her and submits himself to her law" (Blanchot, pp. 49–51). If after reading this analysis, one takes Gille and Stengers's reference to nature in Sade seriously, one must face the question of the connection between the unheroic AIDS hero—the scout who explores "life itself"— and *sovereignty*. Is im-pertinent existence (an existence exposed before all positing, an existence that is a limit whose line runs neither straight nor uninterrupted, an existence that is the existence of exposed and originary Being-not-one) the very last form of sovereignty, or does it open this sovereignty to something other that is no longer commensurable with it?

3. Such an interpretation, however, should not be understood as blurring certain traits of the ideology of science and of christology that seem to adhere to the discourse of heroism in Gille and Stengers. Perhaps it is impossible to speak about a hero in a sense that does not involve heroization and thus representation. The hero of "something" recalls the figure of the scientist who experiments with his own body in order to investigate the unknown, as well as the figure of the martyr who gives himself up in order to embody truth. In a talk from 1980, Michel Foucault examines the connection between the "model of martyrdom" and the two actions by means of which one establishes the truth about oneself in Christianity, or by means of which one becomes the subject of a

"manifestation of truth." These two experiences of physical and verbal self-exposure—*exomologesis* and *exagoreusis*, bodily penitence and verbal confession—exemplify the fact that "you will become the subject of the manifestation of truth when and only when you disappear or you destroy yourself as a real body or as a real existence" (Foucault, p. 221).

4. As early as 1984, Avital Ronell analyzed the emergence of AIDS in relation to the third treatise of the *Genealogy of Morals* and in turn tested this treatise against the effects of the epidemic. Her text, which was ahead of its time, bears the title "Queens of the Night: Nietzsche's Antibodies."

5. "The strongest and most active are also the most vulnerable; they are immunodeficient" (Ronell, p. 413).

6. "As little, however, as the separation between subject and object becomes immediately revocable through the claim of thought, just as little is there an immediate unity of theory and practice. Such unity would imitate the false identity of subject and object and would perpetuate the principle of domination that posits identity. It lies in true practice to turn against this principle" (Adorno [3], p. 766).

7. This sentence can be understood in two ways. The object of the verb *to address* might not just be the limited and exclusive public, the gay men who confront AIDS; it also could refer to the difficulties these men face. But since these difficulties are said to be specific and often unique, one may ask whether their exclusive treatment is not an exclusive addressing-oneself-to, an addressing-oneself-to that is exclusively directed to a particular public. We are dealing with an oscillation by which the position of the speaker can be identified on the one hand as the position of the subject, but on the other as the position of the object. This oscillation becomes possible because subject and object can substitute for each other, because the subject identifies himself with the object and vice versa. The oscillation that expresses identification and identity tends to erase the distinction between subject and object.

8. "My gay identity is not to be confused with my HIV status," Gregg Bordowitz says explicitly (Caruth and Keenan, p. 550). In a text which is an enumeration of lapses and is meant to document the betrayal of his own (gay) identity since childhood, Bordowitz represents the connection between the compulsion to confess and the thinking of identity in such an exemplary manner that one could ask whether he does not distance himself from that type of thinking, exposing it to Being-not-

one (see *Documents*, New York, Summer 1993). The greater the faithfulness to identity, the greater the betrayal.

9. "When the ego assumes the features of the object, it is forcing itself, so to speak, upon the id as a love-object. . . . The transformation of object-libido into narcissistic libido which thus takes place obviously implies an abandonment of sexual aims, a desexualization—a kind of sublimation, therefore. Indeed, the question arises, and deserves careful consideration, whether this is not the universal road to sublimation, whether all sublimation does not take place through the mediation of the ego, which begins by changing sexual object-libido into narcissistic libido and then, perhaps, goes on to give it another aim" (Freud [1], p. 30/298). Freud thus establishes the hypothesis that sublimation *in general* goes back to that which, on the basis of his own analysis, can be described as a form of the work of mourning. If sublimation is part of an economical mechanism by means of which one reacts to a loss, if sublimation eventually takes away restraints from the ego and frees it from object attachments, then it contributes to the overcoming of the loss; it helps the ego to overcome melancholia, a melancholic affliction that comes about through the impossibility of transferring the libido onto another object.

Idealization and sublimation are not identical. The latter "has to do with the instinct," the former "with the object." "Idealization is a process that concerns the *object*; by it that object, without any alteration in its nature, is aggrandized and exalted in the subject's mind." In contrast, sublimation "is a process that concerns object-libido and consists in the instinct's directing itself towards an aim other than, and remote from, that of sexual satisfaction" (Freud [2], p. 94/61). Thus one must not throw together the formation of an ideal with the sublimation of the instinct; however, as Freud notes, the ego ideal "demands" such sublimation.

10. Where he discusses academic discourse, Taylor links nihilism to thinkers such as Nietzsche, Foucault, and Derrida. They share this fate with artists and writers such as Marinetti, Artaud, and Bataille. Taylor thus presupposes a horizon of meaning that has a power of disclosure that seems to make any attempt at grounding superfluous. His description, evaluation, even denunciation, is nourished, to be sure, by the naming power of proper names. Perhaps a connection exists between this method, between the naming of names and a paternalistic authoritarian pedagogy, in whose eyes "students," who find themselves "at the

juncture" of "higher" and "popular" cultures, are supposedly particularly susceptible to nihilism (Taylor, p. 61).

11. "A higher spirit, *sent from heaven,* must institute this new religion among us; it will be the last and greatest *work of humankind*" (my emphasis). Not only does this describe the matrix of all mythologies of reason, but also the paradigm of all attempts to create a horizon of meaning that proves to be lasting. Meaning must at the same time be created and given. It must be instituted from "outside" and from "inside" if it is to be more than arbitrariness and heteronomy. Every meaning transcends the consensus on which it may be based, for otherwise it would be arbitrary. But where creation of meaning happens independently of such a consensus it must be considered heteronomy. Only in absolute consensus or in absolute givenness do arbitrariness and heteronomy become the necessity of the one meaning-less meaning.

12. This constitutive uncontrollability of meaning makes it difficult to transform Being-not-one into a meaningful and significant disagreement. Donald Davidson demands such a transformation in order to secure the translatability of one "conceptual scheme" into another. Disagreement is not to be "eliminated," but meaning is to be assigned to it. In other words, it is to be transformed into a "meaningful disagreement." We thus get at a meaningful Being-not-one, at a disagreement that is determined by the will to understand and comprehend, and that can itself be understood and comprehended as a disagreement. The condition for such a disagreement or for such a Being-not-one lies in what Davidson calls "charity"; "charity" is what the will to communication must demand from us: "If we can produce a theory that reconciles charity and the formal conditions for a theory, we have done all that could be done to ensure communication" (Davidson, p. 19).

13. The eroticization of information about safer sex demanded by Watney ([1], 129) cuts both ways—as does the demand for an eroticization of safer sex and the propagation of safe JO parties. It may be a necessary measure for a life-saving change of sexual behavior, *but it always is also* a euphemism for the submission of life to the state and its police. In this it resembles the ideology and surveillance practices in gay sex clubs nowadays in the United States. Although in some of these clubs one must not only leave a name and address but also present identification and formally declare that one will not participate in any risky practices—in some cases the visitor even has to explain at the entrance what safer sex is—they all have in common that a surveillance light, strong or

weak, illuminates the rooms. There is darkness nowhere: such is the limitation and disciplining of sexuality in the time of AIDS. Masseurs for gay men occasionally include in their advertisements that they give a rebate to "PWAs" (People with AIDS): an invitation to identification.

14. The almost fetishistic insistence on the concept of culture shows a behavior that seems only natural; in truth, it is already reactive. Such a behavior is determined by the idea of producing an identity. What is at stake here is a specifically gay culture, which is to be distinguished, delimited, and defended *as a culture.* In an article entitled "How to Have Sax in an Epidemic," Simon Watney discusses a new CD issued by the Pet Shop Boys, a CD which supposedly permits a "meaningful identification." Watney vindicates a certain type of pop music for the *gay youth culture*—like sex, dancing (that is, the "sax") is supposed to "bind [gays] intimately": "Disco music has been at the heart of gay youth culture [is this *gay* youth culture or the culture of gay *youth*?], so it is hardly surprising that pop music has responded to the epidemic far more pragmatically and directly than any other cultural medium" (Watney [2], pp. 8–9). The songs of the Pet Shop Boys allegedly assert the values of "gay life in the 1990's" and instill new courage. They embody the "sense" of gay culture and its (disappeared?) "club scene," which Watney glorifies "as an almost utopian domain of consensual choice and pleasure." Culture, values, democratic consensus, communication: conformism comes to the fore in the uncritical acceptance of these notions, which determine the ideology of western societies in the 1990's and which depend, ultimately, on the fundamental idea of a production of identity. An uncompromising and uncompromised critique of the politics of identity would also have to aim at these notions. The Spanish band Mecano, which has become internationally known, starts a compilation of songs released under the title *Aidalai* with a song about AIDS, about the virus that "sails through love." The *fallo positivo*—the "positive judgment"— leads to the suicide of someone who cannot bear the puritan morals and the deprivation of love imposed upon him. Doesn't all this amount to romanticizing the disease, to an integration of AIDS into the commonplace formed by misunderstood youth, love, and death?

15. However, this does not prevent some activists from turning AIDS into a negative sign of history, into the negative historical sign of homosexuality. AIDS as a negative historical sign of homosexuality makes possible the continuation of a historiography that perceives history as a fight for liberation and assigns to it the meaning of such a fight: "In the

same way that the creation of Israel was an attempt by the Jews to take control of their lives—and by so doing actually withdrawing themselves from those geographical-political areas where they were most hated, while still thinking that they were doing no such thing, so the institution, growth, and proliferation of myriad AIDS organizations has been considered by many gays as a conscious, positive, creative political response, indeed a historic one, to fight against oppression" (Kramer, p. 256). On November 19, 1992, the *New York Times* reported that Israel, like other nations, would not permit the immigration of HIV-positive people and people with AIDS, because the health and life of Israeli citizens must be protected from "a deadly disease." Critics of this measure, which was called "not Jewish" by a member of the Labor Party, pointed out that its effectiveness could not be determined, because it did not "apply to Israelis returning from visits abroad or to tourists staying less than three months" (*New York Times*, Nov. 19, 1992, p. A3). Does the measure taken by the Israeli government affect an analogy based on the idea of geopolitical control and of controlled self-determination?

16. It goes without saying that insisting on the difference of identities, that is, insisting on the fact that there is no uniformly identical public sphere can also be interpreted as a strategy of exclusion. In the interview "The AIDS Crisis Is Not Over," Laura Pinsky describes the way we often relate to people with AIDS: "What people want to say is 'That can't be me.' They want to find things that are different between themselves and that person. 'They didn't take care of themselves, they had a bad attitude, they didn't think positively, etc.' Blame can be a way of putting distance between yourself and someone else with whom you are afraid to identify" (Caruth and Keenan, p. 552).

17. The idea that meaning can be controlled by a comprehensive and exhaustive context is the basis of a protest action of ACT UP activists triggered by the exhibition *People with AIDS,* an exhibition of a series of portraits. "When the photographs were shown at the Museum of Modern Art in the fall of 1988, ACT UP members protested, demanding NO MORE PICTURES WITHOUT CONTEXT. Part of the context excluded from Nixon's pictures, of course, is everything that kills people with AIDS besides a virus—everything that AIDS activists, PWAs among us, are fighting" (Crimp and Rolston, p. 24). If the linkage between a meaning and its context were essential and indissoluble, then both would become one and, in the end, absolute: apotheosis and disappearance of

meaning in absolute context, apotheosis and disappearance of context in absolute meaning.

18. It is at least surprising that Miller, for whom every word is a concealing and therefore relevant word, quotes the passage that motivates the charge of paranoia against Barthes in a reductive English translation. This passage is taken from the preface Barthes wrote for *Tricks*. Miller cites precisely the sentence where Barthes uses the word "impertinent," which is translated into English simply as "irrelevant."

19. The preciousness characteristic of Miller's writings, presumably meant to be the distinguishing feature of his style, is quite on a par with the "intellectualization" of AIDS, the exclusive parading of erudite allusions and names in theoretical reflection. The will to style and "intellectualization" complement each other. By using a method aimed merely at denunciation, a method that allows no thought time to unfold, Miller conceals precisely the decisive question: whether we should not practice a *free* use of tradition, a *pure use* of traditional concepts. Doesn't such a use become possible where Being-not-one makes us advance to the limit of an im-pertinent existence?

20. Is it not such a Being-not-at-one that Judith Butler has in mind when she expresses doubts about the activist politics of identity? "There are still many people (Simon Watney in particular) who think that political activism depends on a very coherent notion of the gay subject. I think he . . . believes the production of a unified, collective subject is necessary for political effectiveness. I'm not at all sure that activism requires a unified queer subject" (Butler, p. 87).

21. If one follows the logic of testimony, with which we are familiar, then one has to say that testimony of the ordinary cannot be given. The instant one gives testimony of the ordinary, one transforms it into the extraordinary, that is, one transforms the everyday into an exception.

22. Heidegger takes up the relationship between history and possibility not only in *Being and Time*, but also in his inaugural lecture, "What is Metaphysics?" This lecture revolves around what Kierkegaard calls the "nothingness of nonbeing." Heidegger is concerned with showing the limits of science, of a scientific project that comprehends and defines its object. He wants to make clear the quasi-structural limitation of scientific endeavor.

In a note in *Being and Time* that refers to Kierkegaard, Heidegger distances himself from the phenomenon of the moment, insofar as it is linked to the ordinary conception of time. Although he says that Kierkegaard "is probably the one who has seen the *existentiell* phenomenon of the moment with the most penetration," he adds that the Danish thinker did not proceed to a successful existential interpretation of it, because he defines the moment "with the help of 'now' and 'eternity'" (Heidegger [1], p. 497*n*/338*n*).

23. For Kierkegaard, the moment is historical through and through. That is, it is the Being-one of becoming and eternity, the entirely historical as the entirely super- or ahistorical. When he conceives this dialectic of the historical and the eternal, Kierkegaard comes close to Hegel. For the speculative philosophy of religion the death of God as "the most complete proof . . . of absolute finitude," that is as total historization, is "the touchstone . . . by which faith is verified." But to the degree that for him faith must never transform itself into knowledge, Kierkegaard does not share the philosophical interpretation of the total historization of the eternal, the interpretation of the death of Christ as "the death of this death itself," as "negation of negation," as "the most thoroughgoing rendering finite," which means precisely a "sublation of natural finitude" (Hegel [3], pp. 465–66/289–93).

24. Independent of the positions of activism, it should be mentioned here that the Night Without Light and the Day Without Art also belong to the public manifestations of mourning and anger in the United States. The Day Without Art is meant to simulate a world which is no longer adorned by the artists among us. Such a world becomes more real every day due to deaths from AIDS (*San Francisco Weekly*, Nov. 25, 1992, p. 24). The aim is to recall the thousands of artists and their creative energy of which this horrible disease robbed us (*San Francisco Sentinel*, Dec. 31, 1992, p. 3). That precisely art must serve for such a manifestation of mourning and anger, that it must serve as a warning signal, that art is identified with an adorning, decorating, idealizing function (even in order to expose this function), shows that the admonishing, enlightening action is not free of a suspicious instrumentalization of the illness and of death. It is not free of a suspect puritanism. The Day Without Art also seems implicitly to turn against the "moment of enjoyment" in art that Adorno stresses, against the fact that art does not immediately serve self-preservation. Art is punished by puritanism for being useless and for being more than "castrated hedonism" can bear. The Fête de la Musique initiated by the French Ministry of Culture and the North

American Day Without Art are the two poles that indicate the hostility of bourgeois society toward art.

25. Impossibility of reflection that thematizes mourning, impossibility of mourning that has reflection as an object.

26. Made possible, tolerated, and endured: in the meantime, we have perhaps already forgotten or suppressed everything that is happening and has been happening. Cf. the posthumously published article by Jeffrey Schmalz, "Whatever Happened to AIDS," *New York Times Magazine*, Nov. 28, 1993, p. 58.

27. "Mourning is regularly the reaction to the loss of a loved person, or to the loss of some abstraction which has taken the place of someone we loved, such as one's country, liberty, an ideal, and so on" (Freud [3], p. 243/197).

28. When the ideal and identity are threatened, the work of mourning becomes virtually an *a priori* of a life that, without identity and without an ideal, is doomed to death. Every homosexual who leads this endangered life finds himself in the situation of one terminally ill, who knows about his sickness and who therefore has to desire to live life to its absolute fullest. But this desire already thwarts the possibility of living life to the fullest. "One can only live fully if one does not try, if one does not have to do so," Michael Musto writes in his column in the *Village Voice* of July 31, 1990. Precisely because the test of reality results in a split, the homosexual must become an activist, or so the activist's argument could go. But how is such a "test of reality" supposed to take place if the destruction of the ideal and of identity simultaneously destroys the identity of the one who does the testing and the unity of the reality to be tested?

The pathos of an almost impossible mourning, expressed in the question of whether one will still find the time for another friend who is about to die, conceals at times, in the guise of sentimentality, a reckless and conformist attitude. This becomes evident in an autobiographical report published in the *New York Times Magazine* on Feb. 9, 1993. The report deals with gay men's lives, scarcely lived in the time of AIDS. Its author, Fenton Johnson, gave it the title "Lucky Fellow." Here is a synopsis: after having no sex for a long time—he is mourning a boyfriend who has died of AIDS—Fenton suddenly encounters the possibility of intercourse again. By turning intercourse into a birthday gift for a friend whose own companion is dying and who has abstained from sex for years himself, lucky Fenton comes by a good conscience, which he seems to need. The aura of melancholy that surrounds him increases desire and simultaneously puts it in the service of a good cause. This desire is not a betrayal; it is a "triumph over fate, time, and memory," because it pays its tribute to them. "Sad and delicious possibility of making love," a promise whose practical consequences are described with precision by Fenton. For he actually takes a shower before the planned intercourse and looks—as would any decent North American gay—for clean Calvin Kleins in the dresser (p. 18)! Mourning and abstention, used for a stylizing of intercourse, are nothing but the mask of conformism.

29. The threat of contagion turns the virus into a murder weapon. The spectrum of problems that thus arises stretches from used needles hidden in the sand of the beach—whether these are real cases or merely rumors—to sexual intercourse with an infected person who is informed about his health status but remains silent about or conceals the infection. The AIDS epidemic itself is often equated with murder, with the negligence of the government or of scientific state institutions (just think of the blood supply scandal in France and other countries!). Conspiratorial policies of intelligence agencies or negligence, irresponsibility, and accidents in research are made responsible for the epidemic. The more power humans have over death, the more powerless they are. The more weighty and opaque the decisions they must make, the higher the risk of having no comprehensive overview. Does not all this point toward a dimension of the non-natural, organized, manufactured death to which the idea of dying before one's time belongs as well? Is not dying before one's time always murder?

30. That the work of mourning is not necessarily a constant becomes clear to one who turns to other forms of faith and views of the world. In his notes on a Buddhist understanding of AIDS, Dean Rolston remarks that "the essence of life and death is not fixed or solid," but "spacious, fluid, and light" (Rolston, p. 25). Where the delimitation of reality undergoes such a fundamental removal of limitations and boundaries, there seems to remain little room for a work of mourning in the sense of a "test of reality." The aporias of mourning in the time of AIDS are described with precision in an article printed in the *New York Times* in Dec. 1992. Doctors and therapists are searching for new forms and rites of mourning: "Dr. Terry Tafoya, a psychologist at the University of Washington, and Dr. Leon McKusick, a psychologist at the University of California at San Francisco, have borrowed mourning rituals from American Indian

culture to help those suffering from multiple loss. Because American Indians had no immunity to European diseases, 92 percent of them died within two generations of their initial contact with the whites, said Dr. Tafoya, an Indian himself" (*New York Times*, Dec. 6, 1992, p. 32).

Chapter 4

1. No *explicitly* theological reference is necessary in order to interpret and legitimize the epidemic as trial or punishment. This becomes clear in the confessional form, in the attempts at "self-discovery" that produce meaning, restore the coherence of life, and virtually return death to its status as "natural." A line of argumentation is also conceivable that adopts insights of social criticism in such a way that they function in the service of the apology for AIDS, that is, in the service of an apology that subjects Being-not-at-one to Being-one with AIDS. Marcuse's thesis of "repressive desublimation," for example, can be reappropriated if it is inserted into a context in which AIDS is viewed as an answer to the predominance of the genital instinct and as a chance for a revalorization of partial instincts and "nonrepressive sublimation." Under such circumstances, a particular comparison that Marcuse makes in *One-Dimensional Man* and that is already problematic because it is overdetermined by a certain concept of nature reads entirely differently: "Compare love-making in a meadow and in an automobile, on a lovers' walk outside the town walls and on a Manhattan street. In the former cases, the environment partakes of and invites libidinal cathexis and tends to be eroticized. Libido transcends beyond the immediate erotogenic zones—a process of nonrepressive sublimation. In contrast, a mechanized environment seems to block such self-transcendence of libido. Impelled in the striving to extend the field of erotic gratification, libido becomes less 'polymorphous,' less capable of eroticism beyond localized sexuality, and the *latter* is intensified" (Marcuse, p. 73). Equally conceivable in this context would be a reactive strategy that combines a critique of the importance of sexuality and a revalorization of friendship in homosexual relationships (think of Foucault's late interviews) with the idea of AIDS as trial or punishment. Such interpretations would have in common that they understand (modern) history as a history of decline and AIDS as a crossroads where the future will be decided—danger and salvation, condemnation or redemption.

2. Can we use the concept of the given in order to mark the "presence" of the virus?

3. In *Being and Time* Heidegger mentions sickness in two further passages. On the one hand, "the nursing of the sick body," along with concern with food and clothing, serves as an example of the behavior of Be-
ing-with, of "solicitude," an expression Heidegger uses as "a term de-
noting an *existentiale*" (Heidegger [1], p. 158/121). But then the ways a
disease appears, the "symptoms of a disease" [*Krankheitserscheinungen*]
are also examples of the concept of appearance *that is different* from the
concept of the phenomenon: "Here one has in mind certain occurrences
in the body which show themselves and as occurrences which show
themselves 'indicate' something which does *not* show itself. The emergence of such occurrences, their showing-themselves, goes together with
the Being present-at-hand of disturbances which do not show themselves. Thus appearance, as the appearance 'of something,' does *not* mean
showing-itself; it means rather the announcing-itself of something which
does not show itself, but which announces itself through something
which does show itself. Appearing is a *not-showing-itself.* But the 'not'
we find here is by no means to be confused with the privative 'not'
which we used in defining the structure of semblance. What appears
does *not* show itself; and anything which, appearing, does not show itself, is also something which can never seem or produce a semblance. All
indications, presentations, symptoms, and symbols have this basic formal structure of appearing, even though they differ among themselves"
(p. 52/29). The phenomenon is the "manifest" or "that which shows itself in itself." Phenomena as Heidegger defines them differ from appearance [*Erscheinung*] and from seeming [*Schein*], which differ from
each other as well; it is their common dependence on the phenomenon
that distinguishes them from it: "Only when the meaning of something
is such that it makes a pretension of showing itself—that is, of being a
phenomenon—*can* it show itself *as* something which it is *not*; only then
can it 'merely look like so-and-so.'" If one follows the logic of Heidegger's argument, there are symptoms of a disease only because the disease
is a phenomenon without being one. How, then, can one understand
diseases "primarily as existential phenomena"? Does one comprehend
sickness in a "primarily existential" and phenomenological way? Does
one comprehend it as proceeding from the ontological structure of existence if one understands it in its difference from and its dependence on
the phenomenon? Something is manifest and a phenomenon because it
shows itself as this something: the phenomenon has the structure of
"something as something"; the understanding of the phenomenon de-

pends on the "as," on the "explicitness of something that is understood" (p. 189/149) and makes manifest by marking the phenomenal manifestness. That one understands the disease, which in its appearances or symptoms does not show itself immediately, as a phenomenon means that one marks the disease as that which is made possible by phenomenality; at the same time, however, it also means that one marks the disease as that which differs from the phenomenon, from the original "as," from the "as" of "something as something." The task, which fundamental ontology assigns to the scientist or to the physician in the time of AIDS, must read: show—understand—the not-showing-itself of the virus; show—understand—it as such; and thus show—understand—the virus as such. The fundamental ontological understanding of AIDS depends on the phenomenalization of the virus.

4. "Man's being-sick" is also mentioned in notes taken during a lecture course on logic that Heidegger taught in the summer of 1934 and that were published recently by Farías. In its published version the "copy of lecture notes" quotes Heidegger as follows: "Mood [*Stimmung*] transposes man into the totality of beings. Mood opens up the range of beings in a primordial way. Take, for example, the mood of annoyance. He [who is annoyed] does not want to listen to anyone; everything is gloomy. The mood [of annoyance] obstructs access to all things in advance, whereas [the mood of] joy renders all things bright and clear and makes us experience them as we otherwise, in the indifference of attunement, do not experience them. A mood is not present-at-hand in the subject; rather, man is in a mood and by virtue of it is exposed to Being, which mood opens and closes to us [an argument against all idealisms—author's note]. *By virtue of mood we are exposed to and placed in the midst of beings—mood has the force of exposing us to and placing us in the midst of beings.* We are never detached to begin with; we are always already in a mood, and this 'inner,' as we like to call it, is *outside*, and by virtue of it we are outside. The part of us that is visible from outside, the *body*, is the truly tangible and concrete part of a present-at-hand human being. From such a point of view, the body seems to be the supporting ground of man, as opposed to the floating we experience in being-exposed through mood. But if we stand, we do so only because we are *traversed by a mood*; by virtue of a mood the soil keeps, guards, or threatens us [an argument against all materialisms—author's note]. Only a wrong, perverted [sick?—author's note] thinking, which considers that which is 'tangible and concrete' as that which is, will encounter difficul-

ties at this point. This being-supported-by-mood does not dissolve the body, since it is only through its being intertwined with a mood that a body appears to us as something that redeems us or that plagues us. [This is a complication to which we must do justice before abruptly labeling as psychosomatic the notions of sickness and disease we find in the next sentence—author's note.] We say a stomach complaint depresses our spirits, that it affects our mood [*Stimmung*] (cf. stomach upset: *Magenverstimmung*). But, on the other hand, a mood can induce an upset stomach. Man's being-sick is a historical happening of man and is also based on his having-a-mood. Blood, lineage [*Geblüt*], can only be part of the fundamental definition [*Grundbestimmung*] of man if it is defined by that which disposes man to have a mood—his 'mind,' his 'soul,' his 'nature' [*Gemüt*]. The voice [*Stimme*] of the blood arises from the fundamental definition of man, and part of this fundamental definition is that our existence is defined by work, by labor. Work, labor = the present. The present is not that which is now; it is the present as that which transposes our Being into the deliverance of beings—a deliverance of beings that happens in accordance with the work itself. It is as a worker that man is carried away into the disclosedness of beings. As a Being-carried-away-into-the-midst-of-things, this Being-carried-away belongs to the essence of our Being" (Heidegger and Weiss, pp. 98–102). The most important motifs of the passages on sickness and disease that run through *Being and Time* and the *Schelling Lectures*—namely, the motifs of historicality and the having-a-mood or being-attuned of the ill— are assembled in this long quote and complemented by an additional motif—a motif that plays a decisive role in Heidegger's national-socialist texts, the texts most obviously defined by his conception of national socialism. This motif is the motif of work or labor; much later, in a letter to Ernst Jünger, Heidegger comes back to it.

That Farías's edition of the "copy of lecture notes" is prefaced with two sentences that deal with blood lineage and labor points to how little he is interested in reasoning and in a discussion [*Auseinandersetzung*] of the relationship between thinking and politics. His choice is meant to turn the "copy of lecture notes" into a document of accusation before the reader has even had time to become familiar with it. But Farías thus puts himself in an awkward position: it is as if he needs a justification for putting Heidegger on trial. It can certainly not be our concern to minimize or mystify the politics of Heidegger's thinking; we do not want to deny that these politics are meant to be revolutionary in the sense of national socialism. "There is no reaction, because there is, after all, no revolution, because we have not understood what it is we have to attack, what it is we have to do," Heidegger says at the beginning of the course on logic. But we have to be attentive to the text: if Heidegger speaks of the blood that *co*-determines our existence, if he speaks of the voice of the blood immediately after speaking of sickness and disease, he does so in order to trace the discourse of the blood back to *Gemüt*—to our disposition to have a mood. Thus, if we read in a previous passage that the word " 'race' [is], like 'people,' ambiguous and [concerns] that which is related to the blood and body of a people," at least in the context of a people's "life drive and the determination of this drive by the laws of heredity," (p. 24), we have to avoid biologistic reductions. We might conclude that Heidegger's strategy consists of disclosing the "primordial," "originary," "proper," or "authentic" meaning of concepts, idioms, and catchwords of the official ideology of national socialism. This ideology resonates, for example, where Heidegger connects the words "blood" and "soil." The (truly national-socialist) revolution has not happened for Heidegger and will not happen for as long as "being-sick" and all "that which is related to blood" is understood in the sense of biologism.

But what is *Gemüt*? Farías does not even pose the question. In his long preface he does not cite a single passage in Heidegger's work that might give an answer, although he quotes the passage that serves as an epigraph again and says that Heidegger here opens up a perspective "completely unknown in *Being and Time*" (Farías, p. xxxvi). The (putative) evidence of the epigraph is meant to make any commentary superfluous and label such commentary in advance as exculpatory in intent. *Being and Time*, of course, does not leave out *Gemüt*. Fundamental ontology accuses modern philosophy of having forgone a "thematic ontological analytic of the 'mind' [*Gemüt*] such as would take the question of Being as a clue" (Heidegger [1], p. 25). Presumably, Heidegger also alludes to Kant, in whose critique the concept of mind remains unclear, although it proceeds, as is well known, from the notion that our knowledge "springs from two basic sources of mind" [*aus zwei Grundquellen des Gemüts*], from receptivity and from spontaneity. In his book on Kant, Heidegger attempts to ground their unity in the imagination. In his lecture course *What Is Called Thinking?*, he intends to make a contribution to the history of *Gemüt*. " 'Der Gedanc' says as much as the mind, the inner mood, the heart. Thinking in the sense of the word which speaks originally, '*der Gedanc*,' is almost more primordial than

that thinking of the heart which Pascal, centuries later and already in
conscious opposition to mathematical thinking, attempted to retrieve"
(Heidegger [7], p. 139/92). [The first sentence of the preceding quotation is left out of the English translation. In the second sentence,
"Gedanc" is tacitly replaced with the Old-English noun "thanc." Such
changes, however, make Heidegger's point unrecognizable—translators'
note.] Thus, *Gemüt* is meant to manifest itself as "that innermost essence
of man which reaches outward most fully and to the outermost limits,
and so decisively that, rightly thought through, the idea of an inner and
an outer world does not arise" (p. 144/157), any more than mood can be
measured by the opposition between outside and inside in the lectures
on logic.

How does *Gemüt*, the mind, speak, how does the heart speak, how
does the voice of the blood speak in the time of AIDS? Does the virus
expose this voice to a cacophony, a cacophony that does not even form
a negative unity within which it still resonates? How is such exposure
possible? Can the voice of the blood recognize itself in the cacophony
caused by the virus?

Bibliography

Adorno, Theodor W. (1) *Negative Dialectics*. Trans. E. B. Ashton. New York: Seabury Press, 1973.

——. (1) *Negative Dialektik*. Frankfurt am Main: Suhrkamp, 1966.

——. (2) "Sittlichkeit und Kriminaliät." In *Noten zur Literatur* 3: 57–82. Frankfurt am Main: Suhrkamp, 1965.

——. (3) "Marginalien zu Theorie und Praxis." In Rolf Tiedemann, ed., *Gesammelte Schriften*, 10: 759–82. Frankfurt am Main: Suhrkamp, 1977.

Aron, J.-P. *Mon sida*. Paris: Bourgois, 1988.

Bachelier, P. "Moi et mon sida." *Libération*, Nov. 15, 1990.

Barthes, Roland. "Preface" to Renaud Camus, *Tricks*. New York: St. Martin's Press, 1981.

——. " 'Preface' à *Tricks* de Renaud Camus." In Renaud Camus and Roland Barthes, *Le bruissement de la langue*, ed. F. Wahl. Paris: Seuil, 1984.

Bersani, Leo. "Is the Rectum a Grave?" In Douglas Crimp, ed., *AIDS: Cultural Analysis Cultural Activism*, pp. 197–222. Cambridge, Mass.: MIT Press, 1988.

Blanchot, Maurice. *Sade et Restif de la Bretonne*. Paris: Editions Complexe, 1986.

Bounan, M. *Le temps du sida*. Paris: A. M. Métailié, 1990.

Bovenschen, Sylvia. "Progressive Offenbarung." MS 1992.

Butler, Judith. "The Body You Want: Liz Kotz Interviews Judith Butler." *Artforum* 31, no. 1 (Nov. 1992): 82–89.

Camus, Renaud. *Tricks*. Trans. Richard Howard. New York: St. Martin's Press, 1981. [The English translation corresponds to an earlier version of the French text and does not contain the entire text of the 1988 French edition—translators' note.]

———. *Tricks.* Paris: POL, 1988.

Carter, George M. *ACT UP: The AIDS War and Activism.* Westfield, N.J.: Open Media, 1992.

Caruth, Cathy, and Thomas Keenan. " 'The AIDS Crisis Is Not Over': A Conversation with Gregg Bordowitz, Douglas Crimp, and Laura Pinsky." *American Imago* 48, no. 4 (Winter 1991): 539–56.

Crimp, Donald. "Mourning and Militancy." *October* 51 (Winter 1989): 3–18.

Crimp, Donald, and Adam Rolston. *AIDS demo graphics.* Seattle: Bay Press, 1990.

Dannecker, Martin. (1) *Der homosexuelle Mann im Zeichen von Aids.* Hamburg: Ingrid Klein, 1991.

———. (2) "Das ist rein kriminell." Interview with Rosa von Praunheim and Ingrid Mylo. In Volkmar Sigusch, ed., *Aids als Risiko.* Hamburg: Konkret Literatur, 1991.

Davidson, Donald. "On the Very Idea of a Conceptual Scheme." *Proceedings and Addresses of the American Philosophical Association* 47 (1973/74): 5–20.

Deleuze, Gilles. "Mediators." In J. Cary and Sanford Kwinter, eds., *Incorporations.* New York: Zone, 1992. Originally published in *L'autre journal,* Oct. 1985, and reprinted in Gilles Deleuze, *Pourparlers.* Paris: Minuit, 1990.

de Man, Paul. *Allegories of Reading.* New Haven: Yale University Press, 1979.

Derrida, Jacques. (1) "Circumfession." In *Jacques Derrida* (with Geoffrey Bennington). Trans. Geoffrey Bennington. Chicago: University of Chicago Press, 1993.

———. (1) "Circonfession." In *Jacques Derrida* (with Geoffrey Bennington). Paris: Seuil, 1991.

———. (2) "Le sacrifice. Théâtre et philosophie." *Lieux extrêmes* 3 (Summer 1992).

———. (3) " 'Eating Well,' or the Calculation of the Subject." In Elizabeth Weber, ed., *Points . . . : Interviews 1974–1994,* trans. Peggy Kamuf et al., pp. 255–87. Stanford: Stanford University Press, 1995. Translation originally published in *Topoi* 7, no. 2, 1988: 113–21.

———. (3) "Il faut bien manger le sujet." Interview with Jean-Luc

Nancy. *Cahiers Confrontation*, no. 20 (special issue: *Après le sujet qui vient*) (Winter 1989): 91–114. Republished in *Points de suspension, Entretiens*. Paris: Galilée, 1992.

———. (4) "The Rhetoric of Drugs." In Elizabeth Weber, ed., *Points . . . : Interviews 1974–1994*, trans. Peggy Kamuf et al., pp. 228–54. Translation originally published in *differences: a journal of feminist cultural studies* 5, no. 1 (1993): 1–24.

———. (4) "Rhétorique de la drogue." *Autrement* 106 (Apr. 1989): 197–214. Republished in *Points de suspension, Entretiens*. Paris: Galilée, 1992.

———. (5) "Lettre à un ami japonais." In Wlad Godzich, ed., *Psyché: Inventions de l'autre*. Paris: Galilée, 1987.

Esch, Deborah. "Facsimile." In Stephen Andrews, ed., *Facsimile*. Oakville, Ontario: Oakville Galleries, 1991.

Farías, Víctor. "Estudio introductorio." In Martin Heidegger and Helene Weiss, *Lógica. Lecciones de M. Heidegger (semestre verano 1934) en el legado de Helene Weiss*, ed. and trans. Víctor Farías, pp. xi–xlix. Barcelona/Madrid: Anthropos / Ministerio de Educación y Ciencia, 1991.

FitzGerald, Frances. *Cities on a Hill: A Journey through Contemporary American Cultures*. New York: Simon & Schuster, 1986.

Foucault, Michel. "Christianity and Confession." Lecture 2 from "About the Beginning of the Hermeneutics of the Self: Two Lectures at Dartmouth." *Political Theory* 21, no. 2 (May 1993): 198–227.

Freud, Sigmund. (1) "The Ego and the Id." In James Strachey et al., eds. and trans., *The Standard Edition of the Complete Psychological Works of Sigmund Freud*, 19: 12–66. London: Hogarth Press, 1953–74.

———. (1) "Das Ich und das Es." In *Studienausgabe*, 3: 273–330. Frankfurt am Main: Fischer, 1975.

———. (2) "On Narcissism." In James Strachey et al., eds. and trans., *The Standard Edition of the Complete Psychological Works of Sigmund Freud*, 14: 73–102. London: Hogarth Press, 1953–74.

———. (2) "Zur Einführung des Narzißmus." In *Studienausgabe*, 3: 37–68. Frankfurt am Main: Fischer, 1975.

———. (3) "Mourning and Melancholia." In James Strachey et al., eds. and trans., *The Standard Edition of the Complete Psychological Works of Sigmund Freud*, 14: 243–58. London: Hogarth Press, 1953–74.

———. (3) "Trauer und Melancholie." In *Studienausgabe*, 3: 193–212. Frankfurt am Main: Fischer, 1975.

Gille, Didier, and Isabelle Stengers. "Body Fluids." *Art and Text* 26 (Sept.–Nov. 1987). Originally published in *L'autre journal,* Dec. 1985, 10–12.

Green, Julien. *L'expatrié: Journal, 1984–1990.* Paris: Seuil, 1990.

Grmek, Mirko D. *History of AIDS: Emergence and Origin of a Modern Epidemic.* Trans. Russell C. Maulitz and Jacalyn Duffin. Princeton: Princeton University Press, 1990.

——. *Histoire du Sida.* Paris: Payot, 1990.

Guibert, Hervé. (1) *To the Friend Who Did Not Save My Life.* Trans. Linda Coverdale. New York: Atheneum, 1991.

——. (1) *A l'ami qui ne m'a pas sauvé la vie.* Paris: Gallimard, 1990.

——. (2) *The Compassion Protocol.* Trans. James Kirkup. New York: G. Braziller, 1994.

——. (2) *Le protocole compassionnel.* Paris: Gallimard, 1991.

——. (3) *The Man in the Red Hat.* Trans. James Kirkup. London: Quartet Books, 1993.

——. (3) *L'homme au chapeau rouge.* Paris: Gallimard, 1992.

——. (4) *Cytomégalovirus.* Paris: Seuil, 1992.

Hamacher, Werner. "Amphora (Extracts)." In *Assemblage* 20 (1993): 40–41.

Haraway, Donna. "The Biopolitics of Postmodern Bodies: Determinations of Self in Immune System Discourse." *differences: a journal of feminist cultural studies* 1, no. 1 (1989): 3–43.

Hegel, Georg Wilhelm Friedrich. (1a) *Introduction to the Philosophy of History.* Trans. Leo Rauch. Indianapolis: Hackett, 1988. [This version is a translation of the 1840 compilation, which also is the version used in the Suhrkamp edition. Unfortunately, it only contains an excerpt of "The Geographical Basis of History"—translators' note.]

——. (1b) *Lectures on the Philosophy of World History. Introduction: Reason in History.* Trans. H. B. Nisbet. Cambridge, Eng.: Cambridge University Press, 1975. [This version follows the Hoffmeister edition and its significantly different and rearranged structure. We only used this version for passages not contained in the Rauch edition, but we generally preferred Rauch since his arrangement of the text corresponds to the German version used by the author—translators' note.]

——. (1) *Vorlesungen über die Philosophie der Geschichte.* In *Theorie-Werkausgabe,* vol. 12. Frankfurt am Main: Suhrkamp, 1970.

———. (2) *Hegel's Science of Logic.* Trans. A. V. Miller. London: George Allen & Unwin, 1969.

———. (2) *Wissenschaft der Logik.* In *Theorie-Werkausgabe,* vol. 5. Frankfurt am Main: Suhrkamp, 1970.

———. (3) *Lectures on the Philosophy of Religion.* 1-vol. Ed. Peter C. Hodgson; trans. R. F. Brown et al. Berkeley: University of California Press, 1988.

———. (3) *Vorlesungen über die Philosophie der Religion.* In *Theorie-Werkausgabe,* vol. 17. Frankfurt am Main: Suhrkamp, 1970.

Heidegger, Martin. (1) *Being and Time.* Trans. John Macquarrie & Edward Robinson. New York: Harper & Row, 1962.

———. (1) *Sein und Zeit.* Tübingen: Niemeyer, 1979.

———. (2) *Nietzsche Volume IV: Nihilism.* Ed. David Farrell Krell; trans. Frank A. Capuzzi. San Francisco: Harper & Row, 1982.

———. (2) *Nietzsche II.* Pfullingen: Neske, 1961.

———. (3) *The Essence of Reasons: A Bilingual Edition, Incorporating the German Text of "Vom Wesen des Grundes."* Trans. Terence Malick. Evanston, Ill.: Northwestern University Press, 1969.

———. (3) "Vom Wesen des Grundes." In *Wegmarken,* pp. 123–75. Frankfurt am Main: Klostermann, 1976.

———. (4) "The Word of Nietzsche: God Is Dead." In *The Question Concerning Technology and Other Essays,* trans. William Lovitt, pp. 53–112. New York: Harper & Row, 1977.

———. (4) "Nietzsches Wort 'Gott ist tot.'" In *Holzwege,* 2d unchanged ed., pp. 193–247. Frankfurt am Main: Klostermann, 1950.

———. (5) *Beiträge zur Philosophie (Vom Ereignis).* In *Gesamtausgabe,* vol. 65. Frankfurt am Main: Klostermann, 1989.

———. (6) *Schelling's Treatise on the Essence of Human Freedom.* Trans. Joan Stambaugh. Athens, Ohio: Ohio University Press, 1985.

———. (6) *Schellings Abhandlung über das Wesen der Menschlichen Freiheit.* Tübingen: Niemeyer, 1971.

———. (7) *What Is Called Thinking?* Trans. Fred D. Wieck and J. Glenn Gray. New York: Harper & Row, 1968.

———. (7) *Was heißt Denken?* Tübingen: Niemeyer, 1971.

Heidegger, Martin, and Helene Weiss. *Lógica. Lecciones de M. Heidegger (semestre verano 1934) en el legado de Helene Weiss.* Ed. and trans. Víctor Farías. German/Spanish ed. Barcelona/Madrid: Anthropos / Ministerio de Educación y Ciencia, 1991.

Hollinghurst, Alan. *The Swimming-Pool Library.* London: Chatto & Windus, 1988.

Kant, Immanuel. (1) *Prolegomena to Any Future Metaphysics.* Trans. Lewis White Beck. Indianapolis: Liberal Arts Press, 1950.

―――. (1) *Prolegomena zu einer jeden künftigen Metaphysik.* In *Kants Werke, Akademie Textausgabe,* vol. 4. Berlin: de Gruyter, 1968.

―――. (2) *Critique of Pure Reason.* Trans. Norman Kemp Smith. London: Macmillan, 1961.

―――. (2) *Kritik der reinen Vernunft.* Hamburg: Meiner, 1956.

―――. (3) *Reflexionen zur Metaphysik.* In *Gesammelte Schriften,* vol. 18. Berlin and Leipzig: G. Reimer, 1928.

Kearney, R., and J. S. O'Leary, eds. *Heidegger et la question de dieu.* Paris: Grasset, 1980.

Kierkegaard, Søren. *Philosophical Fragments / Johannes Climacus.* Trans. Howard V. Hong and Edna V. Hong. Princeton: Princeton University Press, 1985.

Kramer, Larry. *Reports from the Holocaust: The Making of an AIDS Activist.* New York: St. Martin's Press, 1989.

Leavitt, David. "David Leavitt. Es escritor moral." Interview in *El País semanal* (Madrid), Jan. 28, 1990, 20–25.

Lion, Antoine. "Sida, un combat spirituel?" In *L'homme contaminé: La tormente du sida. Autrement* 130 (May 1992): 170–78.

Marcuse, Herbert. *The One-Dimensional Man.* Boston: Beacon, 1964.

Miller, D. A. (1) "Sontag's Urbanity." *October* 49 (Summer 1989): 91–101.

―――. (2) *Bringing out Roland Barthes.* Berkeley: University of California Press, 1992.

Milner, Jean-Claude. *Constat.* Paris: Seuil, 1992.

Monk, Ray. *Ludwig Wittgenstein: The Duty of Genius.* New York: Penguin, 1990.

Montaigne, Michel de. *Essais.* Book I. Paris: Flammarion, 1969.

―――. *The Complete Essays of Montaigne.* Trans. Donald M. Frame. Stanford: Stanford University Press, 1948.

Nancy, Jean-Luc. (1) "La grande loi." In *Revue internationale de Psychoanalyse* 1 (1992).

―――. (2) "Entretien sur le mal." *Apertura* 5 (1991).

―――. (3) *Une pensée finie.* Paris: Galilée, 1991.

―――. (4) *L'expérience de la liberté.* Paris: Galilée, 1988.

―――. (5) *Corpus.* Paris: A. M. Métailié, 1992.

Nietzsche, Friedrich. (1) *Thus Spoke Zarathustra.* In *The Portable Nietzsche*, trans. Walter Kaufmann, pp. 103–439. New York: Viking, 1965.

————. (1) *Also sprach Zarathustra.* In *Kritische Gesamtausgabe*, ed. G. Colli and M. Montinari, vol. 4. Munich and Berlin: dtv / de Gruyter, 1988.

————. (2) *On the Genealogy of Morals and Ecce Homo.* Trans. Walter Kaufmann and R. J. Hollingdale. New York: Vintage, 1989.

————. (2) *Zur Genealogie der Moral.* In *Kritische Gesamtausgabe*, ed. G. Colli and M. Montinari, vol. 5. Munich and Berlin: dtv / de Gruyter, 1988.

Nixon, Michael, and Bebe Nixon. *People with AIDS.* Boston: D. R. Godine, 1991.

Padgug, Robert A., and Gerald M. Oppenheimer. "Riding the Tiger: AIDS and the Gay Community." In Elizabeth Fee and Daniel M. Fox, eds., *AIDS: The Making of a Chronic Disease*, pp. 245–78. Berkeley: University of California Press, 1992.

Pollak, Michael. *Les homosexuels et le sida: Sociologie d'une épidémie.* Paris: A. M. Métailié, 1988.

Reik, Theodor. "The Compulsion to Confess." In *The Compulsion to Confess*, trans. Norbert Rie, pp. 176–356. New York: Farrar, Straus & Cudahy, 1959.

————. *Geständniszwang und Strafbedürfnis.* Leipzig: Internationaler psychoanalytischer Verlag, 1925.

Rolston, Dean. "Momento Mori: Notes on Buddhism and AIDS." *Tricycle: The Buddhist Review* 1, no. 1 (Fall 1991): 22–25.

Ronnell, Avital. "Queens of the Night: Nietzsche's Antibodies." *Genre* 16, no. 4 (Winter 1983): 405–22.

Schweppenhäuser, Hermann. *Studien über die Heideggersche Sprachtheorie.* Munich: Edition Text & Kritik, 1988.

Seneca. "On the Shortness of Life." In *Moral Essays*, trans. John W. Basore, 2: 286–355. Cambridge, Mass.: Harvard University Press, 1990.

Sontag, Susan. "AIDS and Its Metaphors." In *Illness as Metaphor and AIDS and Its Metaphors*, pp. 89–183. New York: Anchor, 1990.

Starobinski, Jean. *Montaigne in Motion.* Trans. Arthur Goldhammer. Chicago: University of Chicago Press, 1985.

————. *Montaigne en mouvement.* Paris: Gallimard, 1982.

Taylor, Charles. *The Ethics of Authenticity.* Cambridge, Mass.: Harvard University Press, 1992.

144

Bibliography

Treichler, Paula A. (1) "AIDS, Homophobia, and Biomedical Discourse: An Epidemic of Signification." In Douglas Crimp, ed., *AIDS: Cultural Analysis Cultural Activism*, pp. 31–70. Cambridge, Mass.: MIT Press, 1988.

———. (2) "AIDS, Gender, and Biomedical Discourse: Current Contests for Meaning." In Elizabeth Fee and Daniel M. Fox, eds., *AIDS: The Burdens of History*, pp. 190–266. Berkeley: University of California Press, 1988.

Watney, Simon. (1) *Policing Desire: Pornography, AIDS and the Media*. Minneapolis: University of Minnesota Press, 1989.

———. (2) "How to Have Sax in an Epidemic: Simon Watney on the Pet Shop Boys." *Artforum* 32, no. 3 (Nov. 1992): 8–9.

Wittgenstein, Ludwig. (1) *Über Gewißheit / On Certainty*. Bilingual ed. Ed. G. E. M. Anscombe and G. H. von Wright; trans. Denis Paul and G. E. M. Anscombe. New York: Harper & Row, 1972.

———. (2) *Tractatus Logico-Philosophicus*. Bilingual ed. Ed. C. K. Ogden. London: Routledge, 1992.

Zambrano, María. *La confesión: género literario*. Madrid, 1988.

MERIDIAN

Crossing Aesthetics

Library of Congress
Cataloging-in-Publication Data

García Düttmann, Alexander.
[Uneins mit AIDS. English]
At odds with AIDS : thinking and talking about a virus /
Alexander García Düttmann : [translated by Peter Gilgen and
Conrad Scott-Curtis].
    p.   cm. — (Meridian, crossing aesthetics)
ISBN 0-8047-2437-7 (cloth : alk. paper). —
ISBN 0-8047-2438-5 (pbk. : alk. paper)
1. AIDS (Disease)—Philosophy.   2. AIDS (Disease)—Social
aspects.   I. Title.   II. Series: Meridian (Stanford, Calif.)
RA644.A25G36813   1966
616.97'92'001—dc20   96-14817   CIP

♾ This book is printed on acid-free paper

Original printing 1996

Last figure below indicates year of this printing

05   04   03   02   01   00   99   98   97   96